THE DEMENTIA CAREGIVER'S TOOLKIT

AN EASY GUIDE TO MANAGE DAILY TASKS, GAIN CLARITY ON DEMENTIA PROGRESSION, AND ENSURE THE CAREGIVER'S EMOTIONAL AND PHYSICAL WELL-BEING

TINA E. BRADLEY

SERENEWISDOM WORKS LLC

In Loving Memory

To my beloved mother, Louise Jones.

This book is dedicated to you, the epitome of selfless love and unwavering strength. Your life was a testament to the true essence of caregiving. From my earliest memories, you were a constant source of comfort and support, tirelessly looking after our family with grace and compassion.

You cared for Grandma throughout my childhood until she passed away in 1977. Your devotion was unwavering, and your heart knew no bounds. In 1980, when Dad was diagnosed with cancer, you once again stepped into the role of caregiver with courage and dedication, standing by his side until he passed in 1981.

Your kindness extended beyond our immediate family. You were always there for those in need, caring for your aunt, your grandfather, and countless others. Your biggest sacrifice came in 1994 when my younger brother fell victim to police brutality, resulting in a brain injury and coma. You devoted yourself to his care for twenty-five years, ensuring he was surrounded by love and comfort until your final days.

During the years my brother was in nursing homes, you became an ombudsman for other patients, advocating tirelessly to ensure they received the best possible care. The nursing homes eventually confessed they couldn't meet your high standards, and you brought him home, where he thrived under your dedicated care.

Your passing in 2019 left a void in our lives, but your legacy of love, strength, and compassion continues to inspire me every day. This book is a tribute to your incredible journey as a caregiver and to the profound impact you had on all of us.

With all my love and gratitude,

Tina E. Bradley

CONTENTS

INTRODUCTION

It's a morning like any other. You wake up from your bed, only to be met with something that absolutely breaks your heart. Your mom looks at you with eyes that don't recognize you. It feels like your heart is breaking—a strong reminder that many people go through tough times dealing with dementia.

Alarming statistics from the Alzheimer's Association (2023) shed light on the reality that one in nine individuals aged 65 and older will face the tough challenges of dementia. It's like a sneaky thief stealing memories and identities, leaving only a part of who they used to be. Caring for someone with dementia means giving a lot, even when they don't know or appreciate it. It's a commitment that takes up much time, energy, and personal well-being for someone who needs more daily help.

Being a caregiver for someone with dementia means giving beyond your limits. It's a selfless act. You pour yourself into the role, even when the person you care for fails to recognize or appreciate you. It's a commitment that surpasses time, energy, and personal well-being—a dedication to someone whose dependence on you grows daily.

But you're not alone. All around the world, millions of caregivers share their struggles, giving their all to care for loved ones dealing with dementia. The World Health Organization says that about 55 million people globally have dementia, with more than half in lower-income countries. Every year, nearly 10 million new cases come up, making dementia a big problem for older people. Taking care of people with dementia costs a lot—1.3 trillion US dollars worldwide in 2019. Family and friends who care for them dedicate about 26 hours per week.

Dementia not only takes away a person's true self but also hurts the emotions of those who care for them. But there's hope. People who care, researchers, and advocates join together, fighting for a cure, better treatments, and more awareness and support.

I've seen my husband deal with stress, depression, guilt, anger, and frustration as a caregiver. Like many others, he wondered if he was doing enough, feeling the responsibility on his shoulders. We understand the isolation that comes when family and friends stop calling and visiting, leaving you feeling profoundly alone and cut off from the warmth of familiar connections.

Yet hope emerges through resources. Practical communication skills and advocacy help us connect better with loved ones, navigate the complex healthcare system, and fight for better policies.

Have you ever felt like giving up on caregiving? Have you wanted a break, someone to help, or a shoulder to lean on? If so, remember, you're not alone. This book is made just for you.

Are you wondering if there's a better way to cope or if anyone understands? There is. You just have to learn how. This book gives practical tools and tips to make caregiving easier and more rewarding.

Here, there will be templates, checklists, and personal wellness strategies to help you manage the challenges of caregiving. You'll also learn from the experiences of other caregivers who faced similar challenges and found happiness in tough times. This book helps you discover the inner strength to never give up on your loved ones or yourself.

I've been on this caregiving journey with you, feeling the highs and lows, the struggles, and the sorrows. I spent time with my mom, who faced lung cancer, Parkinson's, and dementia. She passed away in 2019. Dementia took a toll when my father-in-law faced it in 2020, affecting my mother-in-law and husband, who became a caregiver.

At 62, caregiving has been a big part of my life. In my teens, I cared for my grandma, a remarkable woman in a wheelchair, with legs amputated and one side paralyzed from a stroke. These experiences shaped my view and made me committed to sharing insights, understanding, and practical help on this caregiving journey.

Even though caregiving for someone with dementia may seem hard, this book is like a life jacket—it gives you the tools and confidence to face challenges head-on.

1

CHARTING THE COURSE THROUGH DEMENTIA

> *There are only four kinds of people in the world. Those who have been caregivers. Those who are currently caregivers. Those who will be caregivers and those who will need a caregiver.*

— ROSALYN CARTER (*100 CAREGIVER QUOTES*, 2020,
PARA. 2)

Caring for someone is an incredibly tough journey. Finding the perfect balance is essential for both your own health and the well-being of the person you're looking after. I won't paint a perfect picture because it's tough, and I feel for you. Yes, there is no denying that it is incredibly rewarding to take care of someone else, especially someone struggling with dementia. But it is also challenging. And it is isolating. However, you are not alone.

I won't throw around words like bravery and hope lightly. Instead, I'm here to show you the raw, unfiltered reality of what it truly means to be there for someone whose entire world is shifting due to dementia. I hope that you'll start feeling a little less isolated. Now, you'll be armed with more strategies and insights to make your life as a caregiver easier.

Yet, through all this, I want you not to lose sight of yourself. You are not just a caregiver; you have your own needs and feelings. You can't pour from an empty cup.

You need to learn how to take a break...and I mean a real break. It may sound simple, but trust me, it takes time to adjust to taking care of your loved one without carrying the weight of guilt and seeking help. Seeking assistance isn't a sign of weakness—it's a powerful yet vulnerable display of strength.

Get ready to roll up your sleeves and dive in! I'm here to support you every step of the way.

INTRODUCTION TO DEMENTIA CAREGIVING

I completely understand the love and concern you feel for your loved one navigating dementia. Your desire to ensure their comfort and happiness comes straight from the heart. Your role in their life is extraordinary, even if they don't always express it verbally—they cherish you more than you might realize.

Navigating this journey with your loved one, alongside doctors and fellow caregivers, can feel like a tough climb up a steep hill. It's completely okay to feel frustrated or even angry at times. Just remember, you're giving it your all, and it's crucial to prioritize your own well-being as well.

Did you know approximately 43.5 million caregivers have provided unpaid care to an adult or child in the last 12 months? That's a staggering number, highlighting the immense dedication and love caregivers like you pour into their roles (*Caregiver statistics: Demographics*, 2016, para. 3). You're part of a vast community of caregivers who understand the challenges and rewards of caregiving.

Being a caregiver has this incredible power to "change your perspective on life" (Robinson et al., 2018, para. 8) and "make you feel needed and valued, adding structure and meaning to your life" (Robinson et al., 2018, para. 9). Learning new skills and coping techniques can boost your confidence and make you a super problem-solver. Plus, sharing caregiving duties can create chances to bond with family, even when things get tough.

In the beginning, your role might involve helping your loved one come to terms with their diagnosis, planning for the future, and encouraging them to stay active and engaged (Robinson et al., 2018, para. 13). This shows your extraordinary power in keeping them motivated for happiness and health.

Thinking about the future might seem overwhelming, but it's a way to honor your loved one's wishes and keep their dignity intact. Those conversations keep the peace, knowing everyone is on the same page.

In this journey, you will feel all sorts of emotions, from the highest highs to the lowest lows. Because, you know what? "Caregiving is a pure expression of love" (Robinson et al., 2018, para. 7). The love, compassion, and gratitude you feel for your loved one will grow, and you'll appreciate every opportunity to be there for them. But hey, stress, anxiety, and sadness are also part of the ride. It's super important to know that these emotions are normal, and you should let yourself express them while seeking support.

And guess what? You've got various forms of support to turn to. Joining a dementia caregiver's fellowship can connect you with others who've been through similar experiences. Chatting with trusted friends and family, who are always there for you, can provide the extra support you need. "If you share caregiving responsibilities with family members, you'll have more time to bond with one another. Even the physically and emotionally challenging situations allow you to learn about, connect with, and support your loved ones" (Robinson et al., 2018, para. 11).

Being a dementia caregiver is an emotional journey that can bring about some profound changes in your life. Remember, you're doing a fantastic job and should be really proud of yourself.

TYPES OF DEMENTIA

What exactly is dementia? We hear that term thrown around a lot. It is a catch-all term for several diseases that pose different challenges with thinking and memory.

And you know what? Dementia can and will eventually make everyday things like talking, dressing, or cooking tricky for the person suffering from the illness. As it becomes more serious, understanding the type of dementia your loved one has becomes essential for giving them the best care.

Are you ready to dive into the various types of dementia together?

Alzheimer's Disease

Alzheimer's Disease is the most common form of dementia, characterized by progressive brain damage over time. The core features of Alzheimer's include the development of amyloid plaques and tau tangles in the brain, which lead to the death of brain cells.

- **Amyloid Plaques:** These are deposits of a protein fragment called beta-amyloid that accumulate between the brain's nerve cells. Think of them as blockages that disrupt communication between cells, impairing function and triggering cell death.
- **Tau Tangles:** Tau is a protein that, in a healthy brain, helps support the internal structure of nerve cells. In Alzheimer's, tau proteins twist into abnormal tangles inside cells, leading to the failure of the transport system within cells. This breakdown causes the cells to die.

The combination of amyloid plaques and tau tangles disrupts the normal functioning of brain cells, leading to the symptoms of Alzheimer's, such as memory loss, difficulties with thinking and planning, and changes in personality and behavior. The progression of these symptoms is gradual but ultimately severe, significantly impairing a person's ability to live independently.

The causes of Alzheimer's Disease are believed to be a mix of genetic, environmental, and lifestyle factors. These elements work together to initiate and accelerate brain changes, although the exact mechanism and interplay of these factors are not fully understood.

In essence, Alzheimer's Disease represents a profound challenge to cognitive health, marked by the gradual accumulation of specific proteins that damage the brain's structure and function over time.

Frontotemporal Dementia

Frontotemporal Dementia (FTD) affects the brain, particularly the frontal and temporal lobes, which are crucial for controlling our personality, behavior, and language. This condition leads to a decline in these specific areas, profoundly impacting how a person thinks, acts, and communicates.

- **Personality and Behavior Changes:** As FTD progresses, it can alter a person's personality in significant ways. Someone who was once patient and mild-mannered might become impulsive, indifferent, or socially inappropriate. It's as if the filter or control we have over our actions and reactions starts to malfunction. This change can be bewildering and stressful for both the person with FTD and their loved ones, as the individual may act in ways that are out of character for them.
- **Language and Communication Issues:** FTD can also severely affect the ability to use and understand language, a condition known as aphasia. This isn't just about forgetting words; it can mean a fundamental breakdown in the ability to communicate thoughts or comprehend what others are saying. For some, speaking might become laborious, finding the right words becomes increasingly difficult, and in advanced stages, the person might rely on very basic phrases or even become nonverbal.
- **Cognitive Skills Decline:** While memory might be relatively preserved in the early stages, the ability to plan, organize, and execute tasks deteriorates. This impacts daily living and can make managing finances, household chores, or work responsibilities challenging.

Frontotemporal Dementia typically occurs at a younger age than other dementias, often between 40 and 65. The progression and symptoms can vary significantly from person to person, making early diagnosis challenging. Unlike Alzheimer's, where memory loss is prominent, FTD's hallmark is the profound change in personality and behavior, alongside language difficulties. There's currently no cure for FTD, but treatments focus on managing symptoms and providing support and strategies to navigate the changes it brings.

Lewy Body Dementia

Lewy Body Dementia (LBD) involves the buildup of abnormal protein deposits, known as Lewy bodies, inside brain cells. These deposits interfere with the normal functioning of the brain in several key ways:

- **Thinking and Cognition:** The accumulation of Lewy bodies significantly affects cognitive functions. This means people with LBD may find it hard to focus, think clearly, or remember things. It's as if the brain's ability to process and retrieve information is slowed down or blocked, leading to confusion and memory loss.
- **Movement:** The presence of Lewy bodies in certain areas of the brain also impacts physical movement. Individuals might experience stiffness, shakiness, and difficulty with balance and coordination, similar to symptoms seen in Parkinson's disease. It's like the signals that tell the body how to move are getting mixed up or lost.
- **Behavior and Mood:** Lewy bodies can lead to changes in behavior and mood. This could manifest as sudden shifts in mood, depression, apathy, or even hallucinations. Essentially, the normal regulation of emotions and behaviors becomes disrupted, making it challenging for the person to control or understand their own reactions.
- **Sleep and Alertness:** People with LBD often face problems with sleep, experiencing vivid dreams, acting out dreams physically, or falling asleep during the day. It's as

though the brain can't properly regulate sleep cycles, leading to disrupted rest and alertness.

The critical aspect of LBD is its impact on both cognitive functions and physical movement, making it a particularly challenging form of dementia. Understanding these effects helps in providing appropriate care and support for those affected.

Vascular Dementia

Vascular Dementia is a form of dementia caused by reduced blood flow to the brain. This reduction in blood flow can result from various conditions that either block or narrow the blood vessels, limiting the brain's supply of oxygen and nutrients essential for its functioning. Strokes, or "brain attacks," are a common cause, but any condition that compromises the vascular system can contribute.

Here's a more detailed breakdown of how this happens and its effects:

- **After a Stroke:** When a stroke occurs, it often affects specific areas of the brain responsible for particular functions. Depending on where the stroke happens, it can lead to sudden symptoms such as paralysis on one side of the body or speech difficulties. Over time, if multiple strokes occur or if a stroke affects areas critical for cognitive functions, it can lead to a stepwise decline in cognitive abilities, noticeable as sudden changes that worsen in stages.
- **Chronic Vascular Conditions:** Conditions like high blood pressure, diabetes, high cholesterol, and smoking can gradually damage the blood vessels, leading to

atherosclerosis (hardening and narrowing of the arteries) and other vascular problems. This chronic damage can lead to tiny, often unnoticed, strokes or reduced blood flow throughout the brain, leading to a more gradual but progressive cognitive decline.

The impact on cognitive functions can vary but often includes:

- **Reasoning and Planning:** Individuals may find it challenging to solve problems, plan out tasks, or organize their thoughts effectively.
- **Memory:** While not as immediately impacted as in Alzheimer's disease, memory can suffer, especially the ability to remember recent events or information.
- **Judgment:** Making decisions can become difficult, and individuals may struggle to assess situations accurately.
- **Speed of Thought Processes:** The brain's ability to process information quickly and efficiently declines, leading to slower thinking and reaction times.

Symptoms of vascular dementia can appear suddenly following a stroke or gradually as a result of ongoing vascular damage. The progression of the disease can be uneven, with periods of stability interspersed with sudden declines, reflecting the nature of the vascular issues causing the brain damage.

Managing risk factors for stroke and cardiovascular disease is a critical part of preventing or slowing the progression of vascular dementia. This includes controlling high blood pressure, managing diabetes, quitting smoking, maintaining a healthy diet, and staying physically active.

Creutzfeldt-Jakob Disease

Creutzfeldt-Jakob Disease (CJD) is considered a form of dementia, although it is quite distinct from more common types like Alzheimer's Disease or vascular dementia. CJD is a rare, degenerative, invariably fatal brain disorder affecting about one in one million people per year worldwide.

CJD progresses rapidly, typically causing severe dementia and a range of neurological symptoms. Here's a brief overview:

- **Rapid Cognitive Decline**: Unlike other dementias that progress over the years, CJD causes rapid loss of mental functioning, often within months. This includes memory loss, impaired thinking, and confusion, which are hallmark symptoms of dementia.
- **Neurological Symptoms:** People with CJD also experience muscle stiffness, twitching, and weakness. As the disease progresses, individuals may develop severe physical and mental impairment.
- **Causes:** CJD is caused by misfolded proteins called prions, which lead to the formation of abnormal holes in the brain, resulting in brain damage and the characteristic symptoms of the disease.
- **Transmission:** Most cases of CJD are sporadic, meaning they arise spontaneously without a known cause. A small percentage of cases are hereditary, passed down in families. Another form, known as variant CJD (vCJD), is linked to consuming meat from cattle affected by Bovine Spongiform Encephalopathy (BSE), also known as "mad cow disease."
- **Diagnosis and Treatment:** Diagnosis is challenging and often involves multiple tests, including neurological

exams, brain scans, and sometimes brain biopsy. There is currently no cure for CJD, and treatment focuses on relieving symptoms and providing supportive care.

Given its rapid progression and severe impact on cognitive and neurological function, CJD is indeed considered a form of dementia, albeit a very rare and aggressive one.

Wernicke-Korsakoff Syndrome

Wernicke-Korsakoff Syndrome is a complex brain disorder that arises from a deficiency in thiamine (vitamin B1). It's often associated with excessive alcohol consumption, but it can also result from malnutrition, certain medical conditions, and absorption issues. This syndrome is actually a combination of two separate conditions that can occur together: Wernicke's encephalopathy and Korsakoff's psychosis.

Wernicke's Encephalopathy

This is the acute phase, characterized by:

- **Confusion and disorientation:** Difficulty forming clear thoughts or focusing.
- **Ataxia:** A lack of muscle coordination, leading to shaky movements and unsteady gait.
- **Ophthalmoplegia:** This involves weakness or paralysis of the eye muscles, which can result in double vision or difficulty moving the eyes.

These symptoms of Wernicke's encephalopathy can be life-threatening but are often reversible with prompt thiamine treatment. The key is early recognition and administration of thiamine to prevent the progression to Korsakoff's psychosis.

Korsakoff's Psychosis

If Wernicke's encephalopathy is not adequately treated, it can progress to Korsakoff's psychosis, a more chronic and debilitating condition characterized by:

- **Severe Memory Problems:** Unlike typical memory loss associated with other dementias, individuals with Korsakoff's psychosis may have specific difficulty in forming new memories and learning new information. There's also a tendency to make up information (confabulation) to fill memory gaps.
- **Cognitive Difficulties:** Problems with concentration, attention, and executive function.
- **Executive Function:** This includes problems with planning, organizing, carrying out tasks, and making judgments.

While some symptoms of Wernicke's encephalopathy can improve with treatment, the cognitive damage from Korsakoff's psychosis is often permanent. Managing Wernicke-Korsakoff Syndrome focuses on long-term thiamine supplementation, abstaining from alcohol, and supportive care to manage symptoms.

Thiamine is vital for brain function, and its deficiency can lead to serious brain damage. The body does not store much thiamine, so it needs to be replenished regularly through diet. Foods rich in thiamine include whole grains, legumes, nuts, and meats.

Addressing the Underlying Causes

It's crucial to address the underlying causes of thiamine deficiency:

Alcoholism: Alcohol can interfere with thiamine absorption and metabolism. Reducing alcohol intake and seeking treatment for alcoholism are important steps.

Dietary Improvements: Ensuring a diet that provides sufficient thiamine is essential, especially for individuals at risk of malnutrition.

Medical Treatment: For conditions that affect nutrient absorption, appropriate medical management is necessary.

Wernicke-Korsakoff Syndrome is considered a type of alcohol-related brain damage but can also be viewed within the spectrum of dementia, especially considering its profound impact on memory, cognitive functions, and daily living activities. However, unlike more traditional dementias, its primary cause (thiamine deficiency) is well-understood, and early intervention can prevent progression or improve symptoms, highlighting the importance of nutrition in brain health.

Mixed Dementia

Mixed Dementia refers to a condition where an individual exhibits characteristics and symptoms of more than one type of dementia at the same time. The most common combination involves Alzheimer's disease and vascular dementia, but it can include other types as well, such as Lewy body dementia. This overlap means the brain is experiencing multiple types of damage, leading to a complex presentation of symptoms that can vary significantly from person to person.

How Mixed Dementia Occurs

Alzheimer's Component: In Alzheimer's disease, the brain accumulates amyloid plaques and tau tangles, leading to nerve cell death and brain tissue loss. This affects memory, language, and thinking skills.

Vascular Component: Vascular dementia arises from reduced blood flow to the brain, which can occur due to stroke or other vascular conditions. This primarily impacts reasoning, planning, and judgment abilities.

Other Types: If Lewy body dementia is also a component, one might see additional symptoms such as fluctuating cognitive abilities, visual hallucinations, and physical symptoms similar to Parkinson's disease.

Symptoms and Diagnosis

Symptoms of mixed dementia can be more varied and sometimes more severe than what's typically seen in any single type of dementia due to the combined brain damage. Diagnosing mixed dementia can be challenging, as it requires identifying signs of multiple types of brain pathology. Often, the diagnosis is fully understood only after examining the brain during an autopsy.

Impact and Management

Cognitive and Physical Symptoms: Individuals may experience a broader range of symptoms, including memory loss, difficulty with complex tasks, impaired judgment, and changes in movement or balance.

Treatment and Care: Managing mixed dementia involves addressing each type of dementia present. This can include medications to help manage symptoms, lifestyle changes to support brain health, and strategies to manage cardiovascular risk factors.

Support Needs: Given the complexity of symptoms, individuals with mixed dementia might require a more tailored approach to care. This includes support for daily activities, cognitive therapy, and physical therapy to maintain mobility and function.

Understanding Mixed Dementia

Recognizing that someone has mixed dementia helps families and caregivers understand why the person might be experiencing a wide range of symptoms. It underscores the importance of comprehensive care strategies that address both cognitive symptoms and physical health, aiming to improve or maintain quality of life as much as possible. The multifaceted nature of mixed dementia also highlights the need for ongoing research to better understand how these different types of brain damage interact and how best to treat them.

Normal Pressure Hydrocephalus (NPH) and Huntington's Disease can both lead to dementia-like symptoms, although they are distinct from more traditional forms of dementia, such as Alzheimer's disease or vascular dementia. Each has unique causes and pathways that lead to the impairment of cognitive functions.

Normal Pressure Hydrocephalus (NPH)

NPH is a condition characterized by an accumulation of cerebrospinal fluid (CSF) in the brain's ventricles, which can lead to an enlargement of these spaces and increased pressure on the brain tissue despite the pressure of the CSF being "normal." This pressure can damage brain tissues and cause symptoms that resemble those of dementia, including:

- **Gait Disturbance:** One of the hallmark symptoms of NPH is difficulty walking, which is described as a magnetic gait in which the feet seem to be stuck to the floor.
- **Cognitive Impairment:** People with NPH may experience memory loss, difficulty concentrating, and changes in personality or behavior, similar to dementia.
- **Urinary Incontinence:** This symptom often occurs as the condition progresses and can include a frequent urge to urinate or difficulty controlling urination.
- **Mood Changes:** Fluctuations in mood, including depression, irritability, or apathy.
- **Headache:** Persistent or recurrent headaches, often worse in the morning.

The cause of NPH can be difficult to determine, but it can result from head injuries, infections, surgeries, or subarachnoid hemorrhage. Treatment often involves surgically implanting a shunt in the brain to drain excess CSF and relieve pressure. If diagnosed and treated early, many of the symptoms of NPH can be reversed or improved.

Huntington's Disease

Huntington's Disease is a genetic disorder caused by a mutation in a single gene. It leads to the progressive breakdown of nerve cells in the brain, affecting an individual's functional abilities and resulting in movement, cognitive, and psychiatric disorders. Huntington's Disease symptoms can include:

- **Movement Disorders:** These include involuntary jerking or writhing movements (chorea) and muscle problems, such as rigidity or muscle contracture (dystonia). Jerky, uncontrollable movements of the arms, legs, face, or torso.

- **Cognitive Decline:** Huntington's can cause a gradual decline in thinking and reasoning skills, including memory, planning, judgment, and the ability to focus on tasks.
- **Psychiatric Symptoms:** Mood swings, depression, irritability, and changes in personality are common in people with Huntington's Disease.
- **Speech Changes:** Slurred speech, difficulty articulating words, or changes in voice tone.

Huntington's Disease is hereditary, with a 50% chance of passing the affected gene from an affected parent to a child. There is currently no cure for Huntington's, but treatment can help manage symptoms. The progression of the disease includes a gradual decline in cognitive and physical abilities, eventually leading to a state that is similar to dementia.

Each type of dementia may be influenced by different causes, including genetics, brain injury, and lifestyle factors such as cardiovascular health.

These descriptions aim to convey the distinct features and challenges associated with each type of dementia, providing a basis for understanding their impact on individuals and families. Research and medical understanding continue to evolve, offering hope for better treatments and ultimately, cures for these conditions.

STAGES OF DEMENTIA

Dementia is a unique journey for each person. It progresses at different speeds. It has three stages: pre-dementia, moderate, and severe, each with its own set of challenges. "Specific types of dementias—including Alzheimer's disease and vascular, Lewy body, and frontotemporal dementia—advance at unique rates and differ from person to person" (Hallstrom, 2022, para. 2).

Dementia can surprise you. Your loved one might struggle to recognize familiar faces or remember things they just heard. Their memory is playing tricks, hiding and revealing things randomly. Their overall sharpness might decrease. They might also regularly miss appointments or even get confused with ordinary tasks.

It might be tempting to think it's just a normal part of aging, but there's a real chance that something might be wrong. It's essential to know the signs of all stages of dementia. As pointed out, "About 40% of people aged 65 or older have age-associated memory impairment—in the United States, about 16 million people...only about 1% of them will progress to dementia each year" (Hallstrom, 2022, para. 10).

Cognitive ability, sometimes called general intelligence (g), is essential for human adaptation and survival. It includes the capacity to "reason, plan, solve problems, think abstractly, comprehend complex ideas, learn quickly, and learn from experience" (Gottfredson, 1997, p. 13).

If you recognize any of the following signs, you should take your loved one to a doctor:

Pre- or Early-Stage Dementia

Pre- or early-stage dementia refers to the initial phase of cognitive decline that is more than what might be expected for a person's age but not severe enough to interfere significantly with daily life. This stage is crucial for identifying the potential onset of dementia, as early detection can lead to interventions that may slow the progression of the disease. Let's break down the key aspects of pre- or early-stage dementia:

Characteristics of Pre- or Early-Stage Dementia:

- **Mild Memory Loss:** This might include forgetting names or appointments but remembering them later. It's more than the occasional forgetfulness seen in healthy aging.
- **Difficulty with Complex Tasks:** Challenges may arise in planning or organizing events, managing finances, or following complex instructions that were previously manageable.
- **Language Problems:** Finding the right words is more challenging than before; may pause more frequently during conversations to recall words or substitute with less specific vocabulary.
- **Changes in Mood and Behavior:** Increased irritability, less patience, or slight changes in personality. There might be a withdrawal from social activities or hobbies previously enjoyed.
- **Orientation Issues:** Minor confusion about dates or times but not losing track of where they are or significant periods.

Importance of Early Detection:

Recognizing these signs early is crucial because it opens the door to interventions that can help manage symptoms and maintain independence longer. Early detection also allows for better planning for the future, addressing legal and financial issues, and making lifestyle changes that may slow cognitive decline.

Management Strategies:

- **Cognitive Stimulation:** Engaging in mentally stimulating activities, like puzzles, reading, or learning new skills, can help keep the mind active.

- **Physical Activity:** Regular exercise has been shown to have a positive impact on brain health.
- **Diet and Nutrition:** A heart-healthy diet, like the Mediterranean diet, may benefit brain health.
- **Social Engagement:** Maintaining social contacts and activities can support emotional health and cognitive function.
- **Medication:** In some cases, medications may be prescribed to address symptoms or slow the progression of cognitive decline.

Pre- or early-stage dementia requires a supportive approach that includes medical treatment, lifestyle adjustments, and possibly modifications to the living environment to ensure safety and support independence. Early intervention and support can make a significant difference in the quality of life for someone experiencing the early signs of dementia.

Moderate- or Middle-Stage Dementia

Moderate or middle-stage dementia, often considered the second stage of the condition, marks a period where symptoms become more pronounced and start to have a greater impact on daily life. This stage can last for several years, and the care needs of the person with dementia will increase as the disease progresses. Here's a closer look at what this stage entails:

Cognitive Changes

- **Worsening Memory Loss:** Memory problems become more significant, extending beyond short-term memory issues. This can include forgetting recent events, personal history, and even the faces of familiar people.

- **Confusion and Disorientation:** Individuals may become confused about where they are, even in familiar settings, or struggle to remember the day, date, or season. Disorientation can lead to wandering or getting lost.
- **Difficulty with Language and Communication:** Finding the right words becomes harder, and following conversations or TV programs can be challenging. There may be a reliance on non-verbal communication or simpler phrases.

Emotional and Behavioral Changes

- **Mood Swings and Irritability:** Fluctuations in mood are common, with individuals becoming easily upset or agitated over minor issues. This can be a source of stress for caregivers and family members.
- **Withdrawal from Social Activities:** As tasks become more challenging, the person might withdraw from hobbies or social gatherings they once enjoyed.
- **Increased Anxiety and Depression:** Feelings of sadness, fear, or loneliness may become more frequent, partly due to the increasing awareness of their cognitive decline.

Physical and Functional Changes

- **Decreased Physical Abilities:** There might be a decline in physical coordination and motor functions, making tasks like dressing, bathing, and eating more challenging.
- **Changes in Sleep Patterns:** Sleep disturbances, including insomnia or sleeping during the day and being awake at night, are common.

Care Needs

- **Assistance with Daily Activities:** Help with personal care, such as bathing, dressing, toileting, and eating, becomes necessary. Safety in the home becomes a priority to prevent falls or injuries.
- **Structured Environment:** You should maintain a routine, and a calm, structured environment can help reduce confusion and agitation.
- **Communication Strategies:** Simplifying language, maintaining eye contact, and using gestures can aid communication. Caregivers should practice patience and find new ways to connect and communicate.

Managing Moderate-Stage Dementia

Management focuses on providing support and adapting care practices to the individual's changing needs. This might include modifying the home environment for safety, using memory aids, and engaging in activities that the person can still enjoy and participate in. Caregiver support is also crucial during this stage, as the physical and emotional demands of caregiving increase.

Moderate-stage dementia requires a compassionate approach, focusing on enhancing the quality of life and maintaining dignity for the person living with dementia. It's a time for your family to come together to support your loved one, making adjustments as needed to keep them comfortable, safe, and engaged.

Severe- or Late-Stage Dementia

Severe or late-stage dementia represents the final phase of this condition, where the impact on cognitive function, physical health, and daily living skills is profound. In this stage, the individual requires constant care and support, as their ability to communicate, recognize loved ones, and perform basic tasks significantly diminishes. Here's a detailed look at the characteristics and care needs associated with severe-stage dementia:

Cognitive and Physical Decline

- **Communication Challenges:** The ability to speak and understand speech may reduce significantly, often leading to non-verbal forms of communication, such as facial expressions or sounds.
- **Loss of Recognition:** Recognizing family members, friends, and even themselves in a mirror becomes difficult or impossible.
- **Mobility Issues:** Many individuals in this stage become unable to walk or move without assistance, and some may become bedbound.
- **Eating and Swallowing Difficulties:** Swallowing problems can make eating and drinking challenging, increasing the risk of choking or developing pneumonia. Nutritional needs may require careful management, possibly including modified diets or feeding assistance.
- **Incontinence:** Control over bladder and bowel functions is typically lost, necessitating routine care to maintain hygiene and comfort.

Behavioral and Emotional Changes

- **Increased Susceptibility to Infections:** The immune system weakens, making infections like pneumonia more common and more serious.
- **Changes in Sleep Patterns:** Sleep disturbances, including increased sleep during the day or restlessness at night, are

common.

- **Agitation and Distress:** While the ability to communicate discomfort decreases, signs of agitation or distress can manifest physically or through behavior.

Care Needs

- **24/7 Care and Supervision:** Constant care is required to manage the needs of someone in the severe stage of dementia, often necessitating professional caregiving support or long-term care facilities.
- **Palliative Care:** Focus shifts towards comfort and quality of life, managing symptoms, and providing palliative care to relieve pain and discomfort.
- **Emotional Support and Presence:** Maintaining a connection through touch, sight, and sound, such as holding hands, playing favorite music, or talking to them, even if they may not respond in the way they used to.

Managing Severe-Stage Dementia

Caring for someone in the severe stage of dementia is about providing compassionate care that respects the individual's dignity and comfort. Decisions regarding medical interventions, end-of-life care, and the use of feeding tubes or other life-sustaining measures require thoughtful discussion with healthcare providers, taking into account the individual's previously expressed wishes and the best interests of their well-being.

This stage is challenging for caregivers and families, who may need to seek additional support and resources to manage their loved one's care while also taking care of their own emotional and physical health. Support groups, counseling, and respite care services can provide crucial support during this time.

Severe-stage dementia underscores the importance of comprehensive care planning, emphasizing comfort, dignity, and the minimization of distress for the individual and support for those caring for them.

EMOTIONAL PREPARATION FOR CAREGIVING

Get ready for a ride on the emotional roller-coaster of caring for someone with dementia! Picture yourself strapped in, zooming through unexpected twists and turns, feeling on top of the world one moment and getting knots in your stomach the next. It's a wild journey, but you've got this.

When the news of a dementia diagnosis hits you like a giant wave, it can feel like you're stuck in the middle of a storm. Accepting this reality might seem impossible at first, but it's a crucial step. Like finding your anchor in a stormy sea, accepting what you can't change gives you the strength to face the challenges ahead with courage and a clear mind.

So, are you ready to take on this roller-coaster ride with resilience and grace? Remember to be kind to yourself, show yourself some love, and lean on others for support when you need it. Together, we can navigate this journey and come out stronger on the other side!

Riding the Waves of Grief, Loss, and Denial

Imagine grief and loss crashing into your life like unexpected visitors, stirring up a whirlwind of emotions after a dementia diagnosis. You're mourning the memories slipping away and grappling with changes in your relationship with your loved one. It's definitely a bumpy ride, but you know what? That's totally normal.

So, let's give ourselves permission to feel all those feelings, whether shedding a tear or letting out a big sigh. Grieving might seem messy, but trust me, it's an important part of our journey toward healing.

Now, here comes denial, trying to sneak in and convince you to ignore the diagnosis or pretend it's not happening. It's a common trick; you're not the only one who falls for it. But here's the truth—facing the reality of dementia head-on is actually a brave move.

Recognizing the diagnosis isn't a sign of weakness; it's a decisive step toward becoming a more informed caregiver. It's like flipping on a light switch to illuminate the path ahead, giving you the strength and knowledge to navigate it with courage and understanding.

Calling in Reinforcements

You're not alone on this ride. There are communities out there, both online and in real life, where caregivers just like you share their experiences and swap tips. One excellent place to connect is the Meaning and Hope Institute. It's like your own cozy corner on the internet, where you can meet others who get what it's like to be on this caregiving adventure.

Don't forget about utilizing professional counseling. Picture having a personal guide right beside you on this. A therapist is like a seasoned pro, helping you navigate the ups and downs. They've got all the coping strategies mapped out, can help you bounce back when things get tough, and provide a safe space for you to let it all out. It's like having a caring friend who knows exactly what you're going through, offering support when you need it most.

Think of sharing your experiences with fellow caregivers, like passing around a virtual box of tissues filled with empathy and understanding. At the Meaning and Hope Institute, you can swap stories, get advice, and find comfort in knowing you're not alone on this journey.

And when it comes to professional counseling, it's more than just talking—it's having a compassionate expert by your side. Your therapist could be that calming voice, guiding you through the twists and turns of your emotions. They're there to give you practical tools and strategies to handle the tough moments.

So, let's make this wild ride a little smoother, okay? Whether you're finding support in the online haven of the Meaning and Hope Institute or seeking guidance from a caring therapist, you've got a support system to help you through.

A Holistic Approach to Emotional Well-Being

Let's recap.

First up, you've got acceptance. Picture this: you're on the first climb of the roller-coaster. Acceptance is like letting go and embracing the ride. It might feel daunting, but it's the key to facing the twists and turns head-on.

Now, navigating grief is part of this roller-coaster journey. It's those moments when you feel the wind rushing through your hair. Grieving is like riding the dips—a necessary part of the experience. Feel the emotions, let them out, and know it's okay. It's all part of the ride.

Facing denial is like that loop-de-loop, that unexpected turn you didn't see coming. Denial might whisper, "This isn't happening," but guess what? You're strong enough to face reality. Embracing the truth is a courageous move on this ride.

And reaching out for support? Well, that's like having a cheering squad by your side. Think of it as a friendly wave to others on the roller-coaster. There are communities out there, both online and offline, where fellow caregivers share stories and tips. They're like fellow riders who've strapped in before and can share their wisdom.

Here's the real magic: within each twist and turn of this roller-coaster lies an opportunity for growth, understanding, and connection. You're not just a rider on this emotional adventure but a fearless pilot. You're steering through the twists and turns with a heart full of love and strength.

Remember, you're not alone in riding this roller-coaster. Many have taken this ride before, and their collective wisdom is a beacon of hope. So, gear up, embrace the adventure, and get ready to provide the compassionate care your loved one needs. You've got this, fearless pilot!

Other ways you can help emotionally prepare yourself, you can:

Educate Yourself

- Learn about dementia and its stages to know what to expect.
- Understanding the condition can reduce uncertainty and anxiety.

Practice Self-Compassion

- Acknowledge that caregiving is challenging, and it's okay to prioritize your well-being.
- Take breaks and engage in activities that bring you joy and relaxation.

Celebrate Small Wins

- Recognize and celebrate small achievements, no matter how minor.
- Focus on the positive moments to boost your and your loved one's spirits.

Be Flexible

- Understand that each day can be different; flexibility is key.
- Adapt your plans and expectations based on the person's changing needs.

BUILDING A CAREGIVER MINDSET

Caregiving demands your physical energy and a strong and compassionate mindset. The good news is that there are many ways to grow your caregiving mindset, even if caring for others doesn't feel natural.

Think of it as developing a superpower, one that's rooted in resilience and compassion. As you navigate this unique journey, consider it a chance to unlock new capabilities within yourself. Let's explore how to cultivate and enrich your caregiver's mindset, making this adventure manageable and deeply rewarding. You're not alone in this; with the right mindset, you'll find the strength and compassion needed for this caregiving expedition. Are you ready to discover the secrets to fostering a resilient and compassionate mindset in your caregiving journey?

To begin to take steps to grow a mindset that fosters positivity and support for both you and your loved one, you can:

Cultivate Patience

- Embrace the understanding that dementia may lead to slower responses and repetitive behaviors.
- Practice patience as a daily tool, allowing yourself the grace to navigate challenges with composure.

Stay Present in the Moment

- Channel your focus into the present, appreciating the moments you share with your loved one.
- Practice mindfulness to stay connected, minimizing distractions and relishing each interaction.

Practice Acceptance

- Recognize that your role as a caregiver will evolve, requiring adaptability.
- Be open to adjusting your caregiving approach based on the changing needs of your loved one.

Develop Resilience

- Cultivate resilience by acknowledging and learning from the tough moments.
- Understand that resilience is a dynamic skill that strengthens with each experience.

Promote Self-Compassion

- Extend kindness to yourself, recognizing that caregiving can be emotionally demanding.
- Embrace the idea that seeking help and taking breaks when necessary is perfectly okay.

Build a Support Network

- Connect with fellow caregivers to share experiences, insights, and advice.

Communication Matters

- Foster open and compassionate communication with healthcare professionals.
- Maintain transparent and patient communication with your loved one, adapting to their unique communication style.

Find Joy in Simple Moments

- Discover joy in everyday activities, infusing positivity into your caregiving routine.

Encourage Independence

- Allow your loved one to maintain a sense of independence in daily tasks when possible.
- Empowering them in small ways enhances their dignity and self-esteem.

Stay Informed

- Stay updated on dementia-related resources, treatments, and support services.
- Knowledge empowers you to make informed decisions and navigate the caregiving journey more effectively.

Celebrate Personal Achievements

- Recognize your growth and accomplishments as a caregiver.
- Celebrate the resilience, strength, and love you bring to the caregiving role.

Practicing Self-Care

Caregivers need to take care of themselves so they can cope with challenges. There is no denying that one of the most important aspects of self-care is getting enough quality sleep every night. When you get enough sleep, it helps you to stay healthy and alert.

Another simple but overlooked aspect of self-care is to eat well and exercise. When you make sure to eat good food, it supports your overall health. Physical activities, especially ones that you enjoy, can boost your mood, which then, in turn, increases your motivation.

Self-care can also take the form of things you enjoy. An excellent place to begin is through calming activities like meditating, reading, and listening to music. These activities promote a more relaxed state of mind, allowing you to see life more positively.

Another critical part of self-care is to care for yourself and set boundaries. It involves setting clear rules for how you conduct yourself. You also need to be able to say no when things are too much and ask for help when needed.

Something as easy as taking deep breaths can become a part of your self-care routine. "Deep breathing techniques done for only 5–10 minutes a day can help recenter the mind. Accompany these exercises with positive affirmations and conscious instruction to get the best results" (H, 2021, para. 11).

There is no denying that daily, positive affirmations can help shape your day. Holding onto positivity can also help you be a better caregiver. "Affirmations can help caregivers feel more centered, in control, and at peace" (Sager, 2022, para. 2).

I want to discuss why caring for ourselves is super important, especially if we're helping others. Being a caregiver can be challenging. Because it's tough on you, it's only natural that there will be times when you will feel unsure, anxious, or sad. It's easy to forget yourself as you care for others, so you must learn that caring for yourself is just as important.

But I also know that you don't have to suffer in silence. Many people and organizations can help you cope with the challenges and stress of caregiving. When my mother felt overwhelmed with the stress of caregiving for my brother, she finally reached out for professional help. I'm glad that she did. It was the best decision she made for herself and my brother.

She also found that many resources and services can support her, from her family and friends to specialized groups like the Anxiety and Depression Association of America and the National Suicide Prevention Lifeline. These have been her lifeline, reminding her that she's not alone. They helped her improve her well-being and peace of mind, improving the quality of life for her and my brother. If you find yourself even beginning to struggle, it's important to reach out before it becomes too late.

REAL STORIES: STARTING THE JOURNEY

Let's discuss caregiving, a journey with tough moments and heartwarming rewards. I have some stories to share from caregivers who've been through it all.

Meet Barbara. Her caregiving adventure began when her son Joel was diagnosed with early-onset Alzheimer's at 40. Barbara and Joel's wife, Cindy, faced the changes in Joel's personality together. They discovered cool ways to connect with him, finding happiness in listening to his voice, celebrating all his achievements, and, most importantly, accepting and loving him no matter what.

Barbara's caregiving role didn't stop with her son; it expanded to her husband, Bob. Over five years, Barbara went from being his helper to his primary caregiver. This shows how important it is to adapt as Alzheimer's progresses.

A game-changer for Barbara was a call from the Alzheimer's Society. This connection made her see that she wasn't alone. Barbara found good communication was key, which helped keep her flexible as her son and husband's needs changed.

Now, let's talk about Ngozi, who's been caring for her father, Felix. She faced many demands and tough emotions. She courageously reached out to the Alzheimer's Society for help. Ngozi points out how important it is to seek support and the importance of special moments of joy and connection. She was emotional when recalling how special it felt when her father recognized her after graduation.

These caregivers share the real-deal challenges of taking care of someone with dementia. They've taught us that there's no one-size-fits-all approach to caregiving. Every story is different, showing us how complex and nuanced this role can be.

Most importantly, these stories remind us of how much caregivers impact the lives of those they care for. Seeking help and taking care of themselves is super important, as well as recognizing that caregivers also need care and support as they handle the ups and downs of caregiving. So, if you're on this caregiving journey, know you're not alone, and your efforts are a special gift of love and human connection!

CLOSING THOUGHTS

You've taken the plunge to equip yourself emotionally and mentally for the vital role of caregiving. These abilities extend beyond mere basics, suitable for both novices and those with experience. No matter how long or little you have cared for someone else, they are good skills for you.

Now, get ready for the next chapter! You will learn how to tackle the everyday stuff of caregiving. You will get tips about managing your time, energy, and resources because, let's face it, you've got a lot on your plate. There will be other practical tips and routine suggestions that can help you better balance your time. Can't wait to share these awesome insights with you!

2

THE CAREGIVER'S DAILY COMPASS

Caregiving often calls us to lean into love we didn't know possible.

— TIA WALKER (*100 CAREGIVER QUOTES*, 2020, PARA 22)

C aring for someone is a profound experience capable of transforming you in ways you might not expect. It's a journey filled with challenges, but let me assure you — it's not just an obligation—it's an opportunity to discover joy and growth.

Caring for a loved one with dementia is undeniably tough. Yet, it holds the unique power to deepen the bond you share. Among the difficulties, invaluable lessons await learning—practical tips that can make each day brighter. From crafting a daily plan to managing your emotions and stress, from speaking kindly to your loved one to finding joy and meaning in your shared moments, you're about to embark on a journey of discovery.

This chapter is like a guidebook, offering insights into navigating each day with purpose and compassion. It's a collection of tools—

how to care for your loved one, care for yourself, and seek support from others. Remember, caring for someone isn't just a task; it's a pathway to personal growth, learning, and a more profound, richer love.

As you dive into these pages, I hope you'll uncover the beauty of this caregiving journey. May it help you face the challenges and find moments of joy and connection with your loved one. You're not alone, and you're not just fulfilling a duty—you're on a path of growth, learning, and love. Let's make every moment count.

STEP-BY-STEP DAILY CARE ROUTINES

Establishing a routine can be incredibly beneficial for both you and your loved one. It provides a sense of familiarity and structure despite the confusion that dementia can bring. While "Learning and short-term memory are typically the first cognitive processes affected by the disease[dementia], habits and memories that are deeply ingrained often fade away last. The repetition involved in adhering to these lifelong routines can help keep seniors oriented, preventing distraction, anxiety, and frustration" (Botek, 2013, para 6).

Engaging in activities they know and enjoy helps maintain their abilities and independence for longer. A routine also reduces their anxiety and frustration, preventing outbursts or feelings of sadness. For us caregivers, it brings a sense of predictability to the day, creating more opportunities for enjoyable interactions and conversations.

Here's a daily plan you could consider following:

Sample Morning Routine

Getting Them Ready for the Day

- Kick off your patient's day by making sure they're clean and dressed. This will bring both freshness and a sense of accomplishment that leads to happiness.

Breakfast Time

- Care for your loved one's body and interact with them by enjoying a healthy breakfast.
- Letting them help you prepare the food can encourage them to feel accomplished.
- Conversations during this meal enhance their emotional well-being, setting a positive tone for the day.

Coffee Chat

- Keep your loved one's mind active and reminisce about good times during a coffee chat.
- This boosts their thinking and nurtures a sense of connection and happiness within.

Take a Break

- Find a quiet moment for yourself and your loved one in the morning.
- Taking a short break allows you to maintain a good pace and avoid feeling too busy.

Chores

- Feel productive by tackling simple tasks around your home together.
- This contributes to a positive mindset and brings a sense of shared responsibility, adding positivity to your morning.

Activity Time

- Start their morning with energy and enthusiasm by adding some activities to kick-start their day.
- This could be simple as gentle exercises to get their body moving or a fun mental activity to keep their mind engaged.

Afternoon Sample Routine

Lunch

- Lunchtime is an opportunity to come together and savor a meal.
- It's more than just filling our stomachs; it's about creating a moment of warmth and enjoyment together.

Outdoors

- Step outside and enjoy the fresh air.
- Whether it's a walk, some light exercise, or just sitting in a green space, spending time outdoors is refreshing and good for your and your loved ones' moods.

Break or Nap

- If you or your loved one is tired, taking a short break or a nap is okay.

Evening

Dinner

- Preparing and enjoying dinner together means working as a team.
- It makes the evening routine more positive and adds to the feeling of accomplishment.

Coffee and Dessert

- Remember your day together over coffee and dessert.
- It's a nice way to end the day, making you feel more connected and sharing stories.

Entertainment

- Relax with activities you enjoy in the evening.

Wind Down

- Before bedtime, do calming things to help you sleep well.
- It's about ensuring your loved one's body and mind feel peaceful and ready for rest.

Paying attention to any signs of boredom, distraction, or irritability from your loved one is crucial throughout the day. Introducing new activities or taking breaks when necessary ensures that your caregiving journey remains fulfilling and purposeful. Remember, the aim is to prioritize your and your loved one's happiness, celebrating each activity's sense of accomplishment.

TOOLS AND CHECKLISTS FOR EVERYDAY USE

Here are some easy-to-use checklists that I've put together to help you with daily care tasks. They can help you keep track of everything you need to do each day. You can copy and print them out or use them as templates to make your own more personalized checklists.

Scan the QR Code to download and print the Daily Routine Template:

Let's make taking care of things a breeze!

Morning Checklist

Help your loved one get out of bed, dress, wash, and brush their teeth.

Make breakfast and assist them with eating if necessary.

Use morning coffee time as a way to have a quick conversation about the day.

Do an activity together such as:

- Give crafting a try,
- Take a trip down memory lane with some old photos or
- Have a chat about an article from the newspaper.

Make sure to take a special moment of reflection in a quiet moment to start your and your loved one's day on the right foot.

Afternoon Checklist

Make lunch and assist them with eating if necessary.

Perform physical activities together, such as

- exercises,
- yoga,
- walks, or
- general stretching.

Complete at least one household chore, such as sweeping, dusting, or organizing.

Together, play a game, enjoy music, or tune in to a beloved TV show.

Set time aside for a break.

Evening Checklist

Make dinner and assist them with eating if necessary.

Set time aside for mentally relaxing activities such as reading, meditating, or praying.

Socialize with family members and friends.

Help them get ready for bed, change into pajamas, brush their teeth, and take care of their toileting needs.

Read a book, say a prayer, or give a hug.

Weekly Medication Chart Template

This template can be used to track the medications that your loved one needs to take regularly. This template covers whether they're taking over-the-counter meds, short-term prescriptions, or long-term treatments.

Here's how it works: You jot down the name of each medication, the dosage, how often it's taken, and the time of day. Then, as your loved one takes each dose, simply check off the box next to it. Easy peasy!

And here's the cool part—you can even jot down notes or reminders at the bottom of the chart, like if they need to take a pill with food or avoid certain activities after taking a specific medication.

With this template by your side, managing your loved one's meds becomes a breeze. It's like having a trusty sidekick to help you stay organized and on top of things.

Scan the QR Code to download and print the Weekly Medication Chart Template:

Please note: The medications below are just an illustration; you should fill the spaces in with your loved ones.

Medication	Vitamin C	Advil	Antibiotic	Probiotic
Dosage				
Frequency				
Time				

Notes:_____

_____

_____

Weekly Appointment Schedule

This template can be used to keep track of your loved ones' appointments with doctors, therapists, or other professionals. You can write each appointment's date, time, location, and purpose and mark it as confirmed or canceled. You can also add notes or reminders at the bottom of the schedule.

Scan the QR Code to download and print the Weekly Appointment Schedule Template:

Date	Time	Location	Purpose	Status
12/4/2023				
12/5/2023				
12/6/2023				
12/7/2023				

Notes:_____

_____

_____

Emergency Contact List Template

Use the following template to list the names, phone numbers, and relationships of the people you or your loved one can call in an emergency. You can also include any medical information that might be relevant, such as allergies, medications, or conditions. You can print out this list and keep it in a visible and accessible place, such as the refrigerator or the bedside table.

Scan the QR Code to download and print the Emergency Contact Template:

Name	Phone number	Relationship	Medical information
John O'Hara	555-1234	Son	Allergic to penicillin
Susan Smith	555-5678	Daughter	Taking blood thinners
Dr. Jonas Johnson	555-4321	Primary Care Physician	N/A
Dr. Mildred Ratchet	555-8765	Cardiologist	N/A
Dr. Phillip Oz	555-5555	Psychologist	N/A
911	911	Emergency Services	N/A

I hope the above templates are helpful for you and your loved one.

INCORPORATING APPS INTO CAREGIVING

As a caregiver, technology can be your ally in providing the best care possible for your loved one. With the right apps, you can simplify tasks, stay organized, and even enhance your loved one's well-being.

Here are some user-friendly apps designed to support caregivers like you:

CareZone

- **Features:** Organize medication schedules, set reminders, store important medical information and track symptoms.
- **Benefit:** Helps you manage your loved one's health effectively and ensures they receive the proper care at the right time.

CaringBridge

- **Features:** Create a personal website to update friends and family about your loved one's health journey, share photos, and receive messages of support.
- **Benefit:** Keeps your support network informed and connected, reducing the need for repetitive updates.

Headspace

- **Features:** Offers guided meditation and mindfulness exercises to manage stress and promote relaxation.
- **Benefit:** Helps you stay mentally and emotionally resilient, even during challenging times.

Lumosity

- **Features:** Provides brain games and exercises to stimulate cognitive function and improve memory.

- **Benefit:** Allows your loved one to engage in enjoyable mental activities while maintaining cognitive abilities.

Mealime

- **Features:** Offers customizable meal plans, recipes, and grocery lists based on dietary preferences and restrictions.
- **Benefit:** Simplifies meal planning and ensures your loved one receives nutritious and delicious meals.

Medisafe

- **Features:** Helps manage medication schedules, sends reminders for doses, and tracks adherence.
- **Benefit:** Reduces the risk of missed doses or medication errors, promoting better health outcomes.

MANAGING PERSONAL CARE AND MEDICATION

Creating a dementia-friendly home environment for your loved one involves thoughtful considerations to ensure their well-being and comfort.

Here are several key strategies:

Reduce Noise and Distractions

- Turn off the television and radio when not in use and be mindful of loud or sudden noises that might startle or confuse them.
- Soft music or natural sounds can create a relaxing atmosphere.

Improve Lighting and Visibility

- Ensure the home is well-lit, eliminating shadows, glare, and reflections that could cause fear or disorientation.
- Utilize natural light and avoid fluorescent or flickering lights.
- Label doors and cupboards with words or pictures to aid your loved one's navigation.

Keep the Home Familiar and Comfortable

- Maintain the arrangement of furniture and familiar objects, avoiding unnecessary changes unless safety is a concern.
- Use personal items like photos and ornaments to evoke happy memories and reinforce their identity.
- Keep the home at a comfortable temperature with soothing colors and patterns.

Make the Home Safe and Accessible

- Install handrails, grab bars, non-slip mats, and sensor lights to prevent falls.
- Secure or remove sharp objects, toxic products, and potential hazards.
- Label hot and cold taps with signs or symbols and consider using a master switch to control the stove.

Use Supportive Aids and Technology

- Explore devices such as medication reminders, blister packs, touch lamps, clocks, calendars, and whiteboards.

- Use GPS trackers, alarms, sensors, and cameras for additional safety measures.

Outdoor Areas

- Ensure outdoor spaces are calming, relaxing, and safe.
- Consider features like raised garden beds, timed watering systems, secured gates, removal of obstacles, and safe storage of chemicals.

Kitchens

- Design the kitchen to be safe and promote independent use.
- Keep the layout familiar, label cupboards, use appliances with safety features, and install a master cut-off switch for the stove.
- Adjust water temperature to prevent scalding.

Living Rooms

- Transform the living room into a space that triggers positive memories and reinforces their identity.
- Create walkways by removing clutter and rearranging furniture.
- Remove unstable or sharp furniture, and cover confusing wallpaper or upholstery.

Creating a Safe and Cozy Space

Personal care for your loved one ensures they feel safe and cozy during these intimate moments.

Here's a rundown of some simple yet effective bathing, dressing, and grooming strategies while keeping both of you happy and secure.

Bathing

- Set a calming atmosphere with soothing music.
- Ensure the water is warm for comfort.
- Respect their privacy during the bathing process.
- Be flexible with timing and methods.
- Watch out for slippery floors and sharp objects.

Dressing

- Offer fewer clothing choices to simplify decisions.
- Organize their wardrobe for easy access.
- Choose clothes with features like Velcro or elastic.
- Involve them in selecting their attire.
- Dress appropriately for the weather and occasion.

Grooming

- Approach grooming tasks with gentleness and patience.
- Use familiar and non-threatening grooming tools.
- Keep an eye out for discomfort or infection risks.
- Respect their personal style preferences.
- Ensure the grooming routine is safe and comfortable.

Dealing With Refusal

Be Patient and Understanding

- Understand that resistance to personal care activities is expected in dementia.
- Stay calm and patient while encouraging them gently.

Provide Choices

- Offer limited choices to give them a sense of control.

Address Underlying Concerns

- Identify any underlying reasons for their refusal, such as fear of water or discomfort with certain grooming tools.
- Addressing these concerns can help alleviate their resistance.

Distract and Redirect

- If they are adamant about refusing, try to distract them with a preferred activity or topic of conversation.
- Redirecting their attention can sometimes make it easier to initiate personal care.

Seek Professional Help

- If refusal persists or becomes challenging to manage, seek advice from healthcare professionals or dementia care specialists.

Respect Their Autonomy

- Ultimately, respect their autonomy and dignity.
- If they continue to refuse despite your efforts, consider alternatives or compromises that prioritize their comfort and well-being.

MANAGING MEDICATION

When caring for someone with dementia, making sure they take their medicines properly is important. Following these tips can make giving or taking medicines easier for you and the person with dementia. It's all about making sure they're safe and comfortable. If you have questions, you can always talk to the pharmacist or the doctor. Remember, they are there to help.

Here are some simple tips to help you do this while keeping their comfort and safety in mind.

Pillboxes and Reminders

- Use a pill organizer to sort the medicines for each day.
- You can also set alarms or use calendars to remind you when to give the medicines.

Keep a List of Medicines

- Write down all the medicines the person takes, including ones the doctor prescribed, over-the-counter pills, vitamins, and anything else.
- Bring this list to all the doctor's appointments so everyone knows what's being taken.

Know Each Medicine

- Learn the name of each medicine, what it's for, and how it should be taken.
- Familiarize yourself with any side effects it might have and if there are any problems with taking it.

Use as Few Medicines as Possible

- Check with the doctor to see if the person needs all the medicines they're taking.
- Sometimes, using fewer medicines is better to avoid problems.

Be Careful With Changes

- Avoid changing medicines, especially during significant changes like moving to a new place.
- People with dementia might find it hard to get used to new things, and changing medicines during these times could make things more confusing or upsetting.

Tips for Refusing to Take Medications

You might often find it challenging to give medications to someone with dementia. It's not uncommon to hear statements from caregivers like, "When I give my mom her medications, she gets angry." Dealing with this situation requires understanding that these behaviors are attempts to communicate. Putting yourself in their shoes can help you see the situation from their perspective and find a solution.

Remember, your loved one's behaviors will change over time, and what works during one stage of dementia may need adjustment as the disease progresses. Stay flexible and open to adapting your approach to suit the person's evolving needs, ensuring they swallow their medicine.

When faced with difficulty getting a person with dementia to take their medication, consider these approaches (*Medication Safety*, 2019):

Break the Process Into Steps

- Resistance to medication may stem from feeling rushed or confused.
- Break the process into simple steps, calmly and compassionately explaining each to your patient.
- Encourage participation in any step they can manage, effectively fostering a sense of control.

Look for Ways to Simplify

- Identify factors triggering resistance.

  ○ Some individuals get distressed by the sight of multiple pill bottles. A solution to this is only to take out the pills you need to give them, keeping the rest out of sight.
  ○ Presenting them with one pill at a time might be effective.

Provide a Calm Environment

- Ensure a calm atmosphere during medication time.
- Turn off the TV, minimize noise, and create a serene environment.
- You also need to maintain a calm demeanor.

Join In

- Make the medication routine a shared experience if possible.
- Take your medications together, turning it into a positive and enjoyable activity.

Rethink the Delivery Method

- If their pills are challenging to swallow, consult the physician or pharmacist about crushable options.
- You could blend crushable pills with foods like applesauce or yogurt.
- Liquid forms are also available for certain medications.

Take a Break

- If all else fails, step back for a few minutes.
- Allow time for everyone to calm down before returning to your medication task after a short break.

TIME MANAGEMENT FOR CAREGIVERS

Creating a solid schedule is crucial for you, especially when life feels overwhelming and time slips away too quickly. A balanced schedule means setting aside moments for you, enjoying activities, and taking well-deserved breaks.

Remember, your own health matters as much as the care you provide to others. It's essential to prioritize your well-being alongside that of your loved ones. Sticking to a balanced schedule and staying flexible ensures you remain strong and capable of giving your best care.

As someone who's walked the caregiver path, I know the struggle of balancing my needs with those of my loved ones. I've witnessed my mother-in-law face the ups and downs of dementia, learning to navigate its challenges. That's why I've crafted a schedule that includes time for self-care, hobbies, and relaxation. I've also discovered the power of prioritizing tasks, seeking help, and relying on your support system.

These time management tips, drawn from my own experiences and insights shared by Morrisette (2023), are here to help you avoid exhaustion, stress, and health issues.

Setting Realistic Goals

- By prioritizing tasks, you can achieve more than tackling everything at once.
- Focus on the most important stuff and see if there are things you can let others help with or do later.

Making Time for Yourself

- Make sure there's a little bit of time just for you every day.
- It is important to do things that make you happy, like reading, taking a short walk, or just relaxing.

Getting Enough Sleep

- Try to get about 8 to 10 hours of good sleep each night.
- Avoid caffeine and screens before bedtime, and make your sleeping space cozy and dark.
- It is essential to take action if you are having difficulty falling or staying asleep.
- See a doctor to discuss effective strategies for managing your sleep issues.

Prioritizing and Delegating Tasks

- Use a planner or an app to track what you need to do.
- If there are things others can help with, like family, friends, or neighbors, don't be shy to ask.
- You can also check out professionals who can help, like nurses or caregivers.

Being Flexible and Adaptable

- If something doesn't go as planned, that's okay.
- Try to find different ways to solve problems.

  ○ For example, if your plans to help your patient bathe don't work out, maybe a quick sponge bath is a good idea.

CLOSING THOUGHTS

But I also know that creating a balanced schedule is not enough. Dementia is a progressive and complex disease that affects not only the memory but also the behavior, mood, and personality of the person you care for. Sometimes, you may feel like you don't recognize them anymore. Sometimes, they act in confusing, frustrating, or frightening ways. How can I deal with these behavioral changes? How can I understand what they are feeling and what they need? How can I communicate with them effectively and respectfully?

These are some of the questions that I will explore in the next chapter. I will share some common behavioral changes that occur in dementia and some of the possible causes and triggers behind them. I will also provide practical tips and strategies for managing and preventing these behaviors and responding to them calmly and compassionately. By understanding and managing behavioral changes, you can improve the quality of life and well-being of both yourself and your loved one.

I hope you found this chapter helpful and informative and realized that you're not alone. Many others are going through the same challenges and experiences as you are. You are doing a great job and deserve to be proud of yourself!

3

UNDERSTANDING AND MANAGING BEHAVIORAL CHANGES

If you can't change your fate, change your attitude.

— AMY TAN (*100 CAREGIVER QUOTES*, 2020, PARA. 16)

Now, it is all about navigating the twists and turns of behavior changes in dementia. It might feel like you're venturing into uncharted waters, but believe me, it's also a chance for you to grow and learn. It can be challenging when your loved ones start acting differently or forgetting things. However, embracing what you can't change and finding the positives in this journey is completely necessary for retaining your sanity.

When it comes to dementia, some common shifts in behavior tend to pop up, like wandering, getting upset, or feeling paranoid. Your mission here is to explore why these things happen and, most importantly, how to improve them. Get ready to uncover some handy tips for handling challenging situations in a way that keeps everyone safe and supported. Plus, we will talk about keeping those lines of communication open and strong.

As we navigate through this chapter, you'll gain a better understanding of the behavior side of dementia and learn how to handle it like a pro. Soon, you'll have a set of strategies and tools in your caregiving toolkit, all geared up to tackle tricky situations with confidence and kindness.

Your focus? It's not just about managing challenges; it's about nurturing love and creating those special moments with your loved one, even when things might seem confusing or different. Are you ready to embark on this journey of knowledge and skill-building?

RECOGNIZING BEHAVIORAL CHANGES IN DEMENTIA

You are on the front lines witnessing the shifts in your loved ones' cognitive functions—memory, language, and judgment—all undergoing change. Your love's behavior, mood, and personality can repeatedly change, creating unique challenges at each stage.

Observation Is Key

- Pay close attention to changes in behavior.
- Regularly observe and document any shifts in actions or reactions.

Common Behavioral Changes

- Recognize common behavioral changes in dementia, such as agitation, aggression, wandering, withdrawal, repetitive actions, or pacing.
- Be aware that each individual may display unique behaviors.

Communication Challenges

- Understand that dementia can affect communication.
- Look for changes in speech patterns, comprehension, or the ability to express needs.
- Examples include difficulty finding the right words, repeating phrases, or following a conversation.

Mood Swings and Emotional Changes

- Note mood swings, increased irritability, or unexplained emotional shifts.
- These changes may indicate underlying challenges associated with dementia.
- Examples include sudden bouts of anger, tearfulness without apparent cause, or heightened anxiety.

Changes in Personal Hygiene

- Be mindful of alterations in personal hygiene habits.
- Difficulty with grooming or dressing may signal cognitive changes.
- Examples include forgetting to bathe, wearing inappropriate clothing for the weather, or neglecting dental care.

Sleep Disturbances

- Watch for disruptions in sleep patterns.
- Insomnia or excessive daytime sleepiness can be indicative of behavioral changes.
- Examples include difficulty falling asleep, frequently waking at night, or wandering during sleep hours.

Agitation and Restlessness

- Recognize signs of agitation or restlessness.
- Identify triggers and potential sources of discomfort.
- Examples include pacing, fidgeting, or being easily upset in unfamiliar environments.

Social Withdrawal

- Be aware of increased social withdrawal.
- Changes in social behavior may signify cognitive decline.
- Examples include avoiding social gatherings, decreased interest in hobbies, or reluctance to talk with others.

Hallucinations or Delusions

- Note any presence of hallucinations or delusions.
- Communicate with healthcare professionals if these behaviors arise.
- Examples include seeing or hearing things that are absent or holding false beliefs.

Changes in Eating Habits

- Loss of appetite, forgetting to eat, or preference for specific foods may indicate behavioral changes.
- Examples include weight loss, refusing meals, or difficulty using utensils.

Aggression or Combative Behavior

- Recognize any signs of aggression or combative behavior.

- This may include verbal or physical aggression towards caregivers or others.
- Examples include yelling, hitting, or expressing anger without apparent cause.

Repetition of Questions or Actions

- Observe repetitive behaviors, such as asking the same questions or performing the same actions.
- This may indicate memory-related challenges and frustration.

Loss of Initiative or Interest

- Note a decline in initiative or interest in activities.
- People with dementia may lose interest in hobbies or activities they once enjoyed.

Difficulty Recognizing Familiar Faces

- Watch for difficulty recognizing familiar faces, including family members and close friends.
- This may lead to social confusion or withdrawal.

Wandering Behavior

- Be alert to wandering behavior, where the person with dementia may aimlessly move around without a clear purpose.
- This can pose safety concerns and may require additional supervision.

Inability to Follow Instructions

- Observe the ability to follow instructions or complete familiar tasks.
- Difficulty in understanding and carrying out simple tasks may be a behavioral change.

Fear or Suspicion

- Recognize expressions of fear or suspicion towards caregivers or the environment.
- This may manifest as paranoia or distrust.

Uncharacteristic Agitation During Personal Care

- Note if there is increased agitation during personal care routines, such as bathing or dressing.
- This may be a response to discomfort or confusion.

Changes in Mobility

- Observe changes in mobility, such as difficulty in walking or an unsteady gait.
- This can impact daily activities and increase the risk of falls.

Loss of Interest in Personal Appearance

- Be aware of a decline in interest in personal appearance, neglecting grooming and hygiene.
- This can be linked to cognitive changes affecting self-awareness.

Keep this in mind: If you spot significant and lasting changes in behavior, reach out to your loved one's doctor. They'll give you a full assessment and the guidance you need. Stay on the lookout for your loved ones!

STRATEGIES FOR HANDLING DIFFICULT BEHAVIORS

Navigating Paranoia With a Personal Touch

Paranoia Challenges

- You might run into suspicion or paranoia; don't take it personally.
- Skip the proving-them-wrong game; acknowledge their feelings and sprinkle some empathy.

Simple Tools as Allies

- Introduce friendly helpers like calendars, clocks, and pictures.
- Hang up a big-date calendar for a daily snapshot.
- Spread clocks around different rooms for easy time-checking.
- Decorate with pictures of family and happy times to trigger good memories.
- Pictures help your loved one recognize familiar faces and moments.

Comfort and Awareness

- These tools create a comfortable atmosphere.

- They keep your loved one in the loop about what's happening.
- It's like giving them a helping hand in navigating their day.

Tackling Incontinence With Compassion

Toilet Routine Essentials

- Set up a toilet routine every two hours or before meals.
- Use signs or pictures to guide them to the bathroom.

Smart Clothing Choices

- Opt for clothing that's easy to remove.
- Consider using appropriate incontinence products.

Fluids Matter

- Monitor water intake, since they may not recognize thirst, with Pedialyte or IV hydration as potential necessary measures.
- Watch out for diuretic drinks like coffee, tea, or alcohol.

Hygiene Is Key

- Keep your loved one clean and dry.
- Prevent skin irritation and infection with mindful care.

Navigating Aggression With Empathy

Root Cause Exploration

- Try to understand why they are being aggressive—
especially if the aggression seems sudden.

Dementia can lead to aggressive behavior in patients for a variety of reasons, both physical and psychological.

Understanding these underlying causes is crucial for managing these situations effectively and compassionately.

Root Causes of Aggression

- **Confusion and/or Fear**

  ○ As dementia progresses, patients often become confused about their surroundings and the people around them.
  ○ This confusion can lead to fear, and aggression can be a defensive response.

Frustration

- Dementia can make it difficult for individuals to communicate their needs and feelings.
- This communication barrier can lead to frustration, which may manifest as aggression.

Physical Discomfort

- Pain, discomfort, or physical illness can cause a person with dementia to act out aggressively.

- They might be unable to articulate their physical ailments due to cognitive decline.

Environmental Factors

- Overstimulating environments with too much noise or activity, or conversely, environments that are too restrictive, can lead to stress and agitation, which may result in aggressive behavior.

Psychological Factors

- Anxiety, depression, and other mental health issues, which are common in dementia patients, can contribute to aggressive behavior.

Previous Personality Traits

- The person's pre-dementia personality might influence their behavior.
- For example, these traits might become more pronounced if someone is naturally more assertive or has a quick temper.

Brain Changes

- Dementia involves changes in the brain that can affect mood and behavior directly.
- Areas of the brain that control inhibition and self-regulation can be damaged, leading to aggressive actions.

Trigger Hunt

- Uncover potential triggers—pain, discomfort, frustration, too much stimulation, or feeling threatened.
- Take a moment to observe and understand what sets off these reactions.

Tackling Triggers

- Once identified, find ways to reduce or eliminate triggers.
- Make the environment more comfortable, ease frustration, or create a calmer atmosphere.

Aggression Intervention

- By addressing these triggers, work towards minimizing or stopping aggression.
- Help your loved one feel more at ease through understanding and proactive solutions.

Decoding Wandering With Compassion

Root Cause Exploration

- Uncover the reasons behind your loved one's wandering—boredom, restlessness, or physical needs.
- Identifying triggers is the key to understanding.

Safe Walking Spaces

- Create a safe and supervised environment for walking.
- Opt for options like a fenced yard or a designated walking path.

Security Measures

- Use locks, alarms, or signs to deter unsupervised exits.
- Consider additional measures like an ID bracelet or GPS device for added safety.

Pattern Recognition

- Pay attention to wandering patterns—specific times of the day or triggered by certain events.
- These patterns might offer insights into the reasons behind the wandering.

Basic Needs Check

- Ensure fundamental needs are met—hunger, thirst, pain, or restroom use.
- Sometimes, wandering can signal unmet needs, so addressing the basics can reduce restlessness.

Physical Comfort Assessment

- Examine if physical discomfort is a factor—pain, ill-fitting clothing or shoes, or side effects from medication.
- Physical issues may contribute to restlessness and wandering, making addressing these concerns crucial.

Agitation

Routine Comfort

- Craft a routine for that sense of security when dealing with agitation.

- Minimize loud noises and excess clutter.

Soothing Activities

- Play soothing music.
- Provide options for either reading or listening to audiobooks.

Empathetic Response

- When they express distress, tap into understanding their emotions.
- Skip the argument game and keep the tone as soothing as your chosen activities.

Repetitive Speech or Actions

Common Dementia Behavior

- Repetition is a familiar companion in dementia.
- Instead of correction, offer reassurance and comfort.

Gentle Guidance

- If questions or actions are on a loop, gently guide them to a new focus.
- Keep them engaged and comforted with tasks or hobbies— occupy their time with warmth.

Remember, the key is patience and adaptability. What works one day might need adjustment the next. Regular communication with healthcare professionals can provide ongoing guidance tailored to the individual's needs.

THE ROLE OF ENVIRONMENT MODIFICATION

You need to better understand your loved one's surroundings and learn how to tweak them to create a safe, comfy, and engaging space for them. A comfortable and safe environment is also necessary for your loved ones as they navigate their behavior changes. Picture this as setting the stage for a positive experience.

Now, let's explore a handful of examples to better understand how we can make these tweaks to the environment:

Labels, Signs, or Pictures

- Stick labels or signs on rooms, drawers, or cabinets.
- Utilize visual cues for independent navigation.
- Facilitate finding items easily and foster a sense of self-sufficiency.
- Reduce frustration and anxiety linked to memory challenges.

Reducing Clutter

- Clear spaces of unnecessary items.
- Prevent tripping and injuries.
- Reduce feelings of confusion and agitation.
- Minimize the risk of fire hazards.
- Ensure essential items are easily visible and accessible.

Adequate Lighting and Contrast

- Illuminate spaces for better visibility and orientation.
- Ensure proper lighting to minimize shadows and glare.

- Help your loved one recognize familiar surroundings and people.
- Avert fear or hallucinations with this simple adjustment.

Meaningful Activities and Social Interaction

- Engage in activities with personal significance.
- Foster social interactions for your loved one.
- Contribute significantly to their well-being.
- Help maintain cognitive function, identity, and dignity.
- Positively impact mood and overall cognitive health.

Creating a Calm Atmosphere

- Minimize noise, distractions, and excessive stimulation.
- Foster a peaceful environment for your loved ones.
- Aid in relaxation and coping with sensory overload.
- Decrease the likelihood of agitation, aggression, and sleep disturbances.

Picture these tools as flexible tools in your caregiving toolkit. Just like a detective on a mission, you'll need to keep a close eye on things and be ready to adjust. Your loved one is on a unique journey, and their needs may change. By regularly checking in and fine-tuning their living space, you're creating a haven that adapts to them, providing the support and comfort they deserve. So, let's explore these strategies and learn how to make them work seamlessly for you and your loved one. It's a bit like being the captain of a ship—navigating with care, making adjustments, and ensuring a smooth journey.

COMMUNICATION TECHNIQUES

Diving into dementia communication can feel like a musical journey with unexpected twists. Words might play hide-and-seek, and frustration could tag along. But fear not because adapting to these changes is your superhero skill, and I'm here to guide you through this unique adventure.

Imagine your loved one's communication is a puzzle, and words decide to take a vacation. It's a bit like a game of charades, but you've got this! Adapting to these shifts becomes your superhero cape in this ever-evolving story.

Now, picture eye contact as your secret handshake. Gazing into your loved one's eyes and using their name creates a cozy haven of familiarity. These non-verbal cues, especially the magic of eye contact, become your communication sidekick, boosting understanding and connection.

But let's not forget tone, volume, and body language—the unsung heroes of effective communication. Your calm, reassuring tone and warm gestures transform the atmosphere into a safe and supportive haven. They're like the background music that sets the perfect tone for your caregiving symphony.

And when words play hard to get, step into the world of non-verbal connection. A gentle touch, a comforting gesture, or simply resting your hand on their shoulder becomes a silent dialogue that speaks volumes when words take a backseat.

But here's the magic—it's not just about your talking. It's a conversation, a mutual exchange. Tune in, my friend, and let your loved one share their thoughts and feelings. It's not a monologue; it's a beautiful duet.

So, as you navigate the twists and turns of this communication adventure, keep tweaking your approach. Your support is the compass guiding your loved ones through the uncharted waters of dementia, especially in those early stages. You're not just communicating; you're orchestrating a symphony of care and connection. You're a true maestro, and I'm here to cheer you on with every note.

Communication in the Early Stage

During the early stages of dementia, your loved one may still be able to participate in meaningful conversation and social activities. However, they may experience memory loss or have difficulty finding the right words. They may also feel overwhelmed by excessive stimulation and tend to repeat stories.

Some tips for communicating with your loved one in the early stage are:

- Don't make assumptions about your loved one's ability to communicate because of the diagnosis. The disease affects each person differently.
- Make time to actively listen to your loved one's thoughts, feelings, and needs.
- Give them time to respond.
- Don't interrupt unless help is requested.
- Ask what the person is comfortable doing and what assistance they may need.
- Talk about which communication style works for them.

  ○ In-person conversations, emails, text, or phone calls.

- Laughter is important. At times, humor can help ease the atmosphere and facilitate communication.
- Don't pull away: Your honesty, friendship, and support are important to the person.

Communication in the Middle Stage

In the middle stage of dementia, which is typically the longest and can last for many years, your loved one will have greater difficulty communicating and will require more direct care.

Some tips for communicating with a person in the middle stage of dementia are:

- Engage your loved one in a quiet space with minimal distractions for a one-on-one conversation.
- It is important to enunciate your words and look directly at the person you are speaking to, as this demonstrates that you are attentive and concerned.
- Be patient and offer reassurance. It may encourage your patient to explain his or her thoughts.
- Ask one question at a time. Ask yes or no questions. An instance of using more straightforward and more direct language would be asking, "Do you feel like sleeping?" instead of "How are you feeling?"
- Offer limited options, for instance, "Hamburger or chicken for lunch?" instead of "What do you want for lunch?"
- Try using different words if someone doesn't understand what you're saying. For instance, if you ask someone if they're hungry and don't respond, you could say, "Dinner is ready now. Let's eat." This will help them understand what you're trying to communicate.
- Try not to say, "Don't you remember?" or "I told you."

- If you become frustrated, take a timeout for yourself.

Communication in the Late Stage

In the late stage of dementia, your loved one may have limited or no verbal communication ability. As their verbal communication skills deteriorate, your loved one may rely increasingly on nonverbal communication. Nonverbal communication is communicating through facial expressions, body language, and sounds.

Remember to be patient with your loved one, as they may also be experiencing changes in sleeping, eating, and toileting. These changes can increase frustration, which in turn affects their ability to communicate clearly.

Some tips for communicating with a person in the late stage are:

- Use all five senses for communication and comfort.
- Be respectful and avoid talking down to them or as if he or she isn't there.
- Play familiar music, sing, or read to them.

  o These activities may stimulate memories and emotions.

- Approach your loved one from the front and identify yourself.

  o Use his or her name and your name.

- Speak calmly and softly. Say what you are going to do before you do it.

  o For instance, you could say, "I'm going to help you get up now."

- Keep communication simple and concrete.

  ○ Don't ask open-ended questions or provide too many choices or instructions.

- Pay attention to their nonverbal cues, such as facial expressions, body movements, and sounds.

  ○ Try to understand what they are feeling and respond accordingly.

Listening and Reassuring

Taking care of someone with dementia is more than just checking off tasks on a list; it's about honing the skill of listening and comforting. It's like becoming a compassionate guide through the journey of their changing world.

Enhancing Listening Skills

Give Undivided Attention

- Put away distractions and make eye contact.

  ○ "I'm here, just for you. No distractions."

- Turn off the TV or radio during conversations.
- Close the door to minimize external noises.

Be Patient With Responses

- Allow extra time and avoid interrupting.

  ○ "Take your time; I'll listen whenever you're ready."

- Use gentle prompts like, "I'm listening whenever you're ready to share."
- Practice deep breathing to maintain a calm and patient demeanor.

Use Non-Verbal Cues

- Nod or provide a reassuring touch.

  ○ "I hear you," with a reassuring nod and smile.

- Mirror their body language to create a sense of connection.
- Place a hand on their arm as a gesture of comfort.

Reflective Listening

- Repeat or paraphrase for understanding.

  ○ "So, if I understand correctly, you're feeling..."

- Summarize what they've said to confirm your understanding.
- Use phrases like, "It sounds like you're saying..."

Developing Reassuring Skills

Offer Comforting Touch

- Give gentle pats or hold hands for reassurance.

  ○ "I'm right here with you, holding your hand."

- Rub their back gently to provide a sense of comfort.
- Offer a hug if they seem open to physical contact.

Choose Calming Words

- Use a soothing tone to keep the language simple.

  ○ "You're safe here; I'm here to help and support you."

- Say, "We'll get through this together; I'm by your side."
- Use phrases like, "I'm here to make things easier for you."

Validate Feelings

- Acknowledge emotions without judgment.

  ○ "It's okay to feel this way; I'm here for you."

- Express empathy by saying, "I can imagine this is tough for you."
- Validate their feelings with phrases like, "Your emotions matter, and I'm here to listen."

Redirect Negative Thoughts

- Shift focus to positive or neutral topics.

  ○ "Let's talk about something that brings you joy. What's your favorite memory?"

- Introduce a favorite hobby or interest to steer away from distressing thoughts.
- Share a light-hearted anecdote or funny story to change the emotional tone.

Create a Calm Environment

- Minimize noise and distractions.

  ○ "Let's find a quieter spot where we can talk without any disturbances."

- Adjust lighting to create a calming atmosphere.
- Use soft background music to promote relaxation.

Repetition With Patience

- Repeat information with patience.

  ○ "I know we've talked about this before, but I'm here to help you as often as you need."

- Reiterate key details calmly without expressing frustration.
- Offer reminders with a reassuring tone, reinforcing a sense of security.

Use Familiar Objects

- Surround them with comforting items.

  ○ "Look at this photo album; it pictures our happy moments together. Remember this one?"

- Introduce cherished objects, like a favorite blanket or a familiar artwork.
- Display family photos or mementos that evoke positive memories.

Remember, these examples are just some of the many tools in your caregiving toolkit. Feel free to adapt and personalize them based on your loved one's preferences and needs. Your compassionate approach will continue to strengthen the connection and support you provide.

Modeled Conversation: The Loved One Is Agitated and Confused

Caregiver (C): (Gently placing a hand on the loved one's shoulder) "Hey there, Mom. I can see that something's on your mind. What's going on?"

Loved One (L): "I... I don't know. Everything is just confusing."

C: (Nodding with understanding) "I get it, Mom. It's okay to feel that way. I'm here to listen. Can you tell me what's confusing you right now?"

L: "I don't remember where we are. And these faces... they feel strange."

C: (Smiling reassuringly) "I understand this place might seem unfamiliar, but we're at home. And these are family photos; these are the people who love you. It's our safe space. How about we sit down and chat about some good memories? Like the time we went on that amazing vacation together."

L: (Looking at the photos) "Oh, yes! I remember that. It was beautiful."

C: (Encouragingly) "Absolutely, Mom! Those were some wonderful times. And guess what? We can relive those moments anytime you want. Now, tell me more about that vacation. What was your favorite part?"

L: (Smiling) "The beach! The sound of the waves was so calming."

C: (Nodding) "The beach was incredible. It's amazing how those memories can bring us peace. If you ever feel confused or unsure, just remember that I'm here to help you find that calmness again. We'll navigate through it together."

L: (Squeezing the caregiver's hand) "Thank you, dear. I appreciate you being here."

C: (Smiling warmly) "Always, Mom. We're a team. Let's create more beautiful moments together, okay?"

Involvement in Decision Making

One way to involve your loved one in decisions about their care is to use the following strategies:

- Provide information and emotional support to help your loved one understand the situation and available options.
- Respect their preferences and choices and involve them in decision-making as much as possible.
- Carry out the agreed action plan and monitor the outcomes and effects of the decision.

- You should review the decision regularly and adjust it based on your patient's changing needs and wishes.

These strategies can help promote your loved one's autonomy and dignity and improve their quality of life and well-being. It can also help you communicate effectively and compassionately with them and avoid conflicts or misunderstandings.

STORIES OF CHALLENGE AND TRIUMPH

Dementia. It's more than just a brain disorder; it's a journey that impacts memory, thinking, and behavior. It's essential to understand that dementia isn't a normal part of aging, and, unfortunately, there's no magic cure for it. Caring for someone with dementia can be a wild ride for anyone. It can be challenging, rewarding, and downright exhausting all at once.

As a caregiver, you're not just handling day-to-day tasks but navigating complex emotional terrain. It demands patience, compassion, and resilience, which may sometimes feel like a superhero cape. Making tough decisions, dealing with emotional stress, and seeking support and resources become a part of your daily routine.

Let's hear from real-life superheroes–four caregivers on this journey with their loved ones battling dementia. Each is at a different point in their caregiving adventure, bringing unique perspectives and approaches. Their stories will shed light on the common issues and challenges caregivers face, sprinkled with strategies and solutions that have helped them along the way.

You're not alone, and a wealth of knowledge and support awaits you.

Eileen and Marie

Meet Eileen and Marie, two incredible caregivers facing the challenges of Alzheimer's, each in their own unique way.

Eileen, a seasoned caregiver, has been on this journey for four years, caring for her husband with memory issues. It's difficult, especially when you're going solo and your adult children and grandkids are miles away. Despite their distant support, Eileen juggled a full-time job she truly loved. Her husband's clear-headed days recently became clouded, leading to challenging moments and debates about Eileen's job and returning him home.

After heartfelt conversations with her kids, Eileen discovered a local place specializing in memory care. Making a tough decision, she moved her husband there, following the advice not to visit for two weeks to help him settle. When the reunion finally happened, emotions ran high, but Eileen and her husband talked it out. She decided to quit her job, bring him home, and savor precious moments together. Eileen's journey highlights the importance of finding the right balance for the caregiver and their loved one.

Now, let's shift our focus to Marie, a newcomer to Alzheimer's caregiving. Her dad's diagnosis last year reshaped the dynamics at home, where she, her husband, and their young daughter live with her parents. Full-time work and numerous responsibilities make this journey even more challenging for Marie.

Acceptance becomes Marie's lesson as she grapples with her changing relationship with her dad. The frustration of missing the father she once knew tugs at her heart. Juggling work, caregiving, and her own family, Marie confronts moments of impatience and guilt. However, through this emotional maze, Marie is learning to embrace the "new normal." She's discovering the art of cherishing the good moments, letting go of the challenging ones, and finding strength in asking for help and prioritizing self-care.

Eileen and Marie's stories unveil the dance of caregiving, where every decision is a labor of love. As we unravel these tales, remember you're not alone in your journey. We're here, sharing, learning, and supporting each other step by step.

Edgar Caring for His Wife

Let's step into Edgar's world, where he's been the anchor for his wife's care journey for a decade. His wife battles dementia, and Edgar, with a humble heart, shares that he's still learning, still figuring it out—no easy feat, but he's navigating it with love and dedication.

A few years back, a tough episode unfolded when his wife had a fall, breaking her thigh bone. Another fall soon followed, leading to a hospital stay with three fractured spine bones. The pain was intense, and doctors prescribed opioid painkillers. Unfortunately, these medications brought unexpected changes to her personality, complicating the recovery journey. From hospital to rehab, the impact lingered.

Edgar, armed with newfound knowledge about opioid side effects, emphasizes the importance of seeking a second opinion before diving into such medications. Cautioning against prolonged use, he advises limiting them to no more than a week. It's a powerful reminder to question, understand, and explore alternatives.

Edgar witnesses different situations in his wife's assisted living facility, each with its challenges. He quickly acknowledges that what works for him might not fit others' circumstances. Still, he passionately raises a warning flag about opioid medications, sharing his journey of keeping his wife's drug use to a minimum.

Edgar's core message revolves around vigilance. If more medication ever becomes necessary, he vows to engage in thoughtful conversations with her doctors, probing about potential side effects and alternative solutions. It's a story of advocacy, of a husband committed to the well-being of his beloved. Remember, in your caregiving journey, each step counts, and your questions matter. You're not alone—we're here, learning and supporting one another.

Sue Caring for Her Husband

Meet Bill Starrs, an engineer extraordinaire at GM, diagnosed with Alzheimer's at 59. Bill, known for his vibrancy, hobbies, and skills, faced a harsh reality. The diagnosis clashed with his dynamic personality and countless achievements. His wife and dedicated caregiver, Sue Starrs, was beside him throughout this challenging journey.

Sue, equipped with insights from her husband's family history and lessons learned from caring for her mother-in-law with dementia, recognized the early signs in Bill. For eleven years, she played the role of caregiver at home and then three more in a memory care facility. Sue wasn't just any caregiver; she was a hospice chaplain, intimately aware of the struggles caregiving entails.

Drawing from her rich experience, Sue shares advice that resonates deeply. She urges fellow caregivers to base decisions on the safety and health of their loved ones and themselves. Sue sounds a warning bell about the behavioral changes Alzheimer's can bring, emphasizing the need for preparation.

In a poignant moment, Sue recounts when Bill, once adept in the kitchen, became confused with boiling water, holding a cup uncertainly. It's a vivid snapshot of the challenges caregivers face in their daily lives.

Tragically, Sue bid farewell to Bill in September 2020 during the throes of the COVID-19 pandemic. The circumstances were heart-wrenching—Sue and her son underwent rapid COVID-19 tests to spend one precious hour with Bill on the day he passed. Living in Michigan, Sue has long supported the Alzheimer's Association, volunteering at the Walk to End Alzheimer's in Wisconsin.

These stories, like Sue and Bill's, echo the universal challenges and lessons of caregiving. Each narrative is a beacon of hope regardless of where you are in your caregiving journey. Research, education, and awareness become powerful tools for caregivers in this collective journey. As we share resources and tips, each caregiver contributes support. Remember, there's always hope—growing, learning, and supporting one another.

CLOSING THOUGHTS

In our last chapter, we tackled the twists and turns of behavioral changes in dementia, arming ourselves with practical strategies to navigate the challenges. But, here's the truth—I see you. I know the toll it takes on you, juggling the care of your loved one and your well-being.

Let's talk about self-care because, my friend, you're not a superhero (though you sure act like one!). Caring for someone with dementia is a marathon, not a sprint—your physical, mental, and emotional well-being matter. They matter a lot.

In our next chapter, we're delving deep into your world. It's all about ensuring your well-being, keeping that resilience intact, and, dare I say, rediscovering some strength within yourself. I've got a bag of tips and resources ready for you—strategies to kick stress to the curb, manage those emotions, seek the support you deserve, and find the elusive balance in your life.

So, grab your metaphorical cape because, my friend, you're the hero of this story. We'll navigate these challenges together, ensuring you're surviving and they're thriving on this caregiving journey. Are you ready? I know you are! Let's dive in!

4

THE CAREGIVER'S SANCTUARY

> *Rest and self-care are so important. When you take time to replenish your spirit, it allows you to serve others from the overflow. You cannot serve from an empty vessel.*
>
> — ELEANOR BROWNN (*100 CAREGIVER QUOTES*, 2020, PARA. 60)

Taking care of yourself isn't just a luxury—it's a necessity. Picture this: you're like a superhero, and self-care is your secret power source. It's not about being selfish; it's about recharging those superhero batteries so you can keep spreading your incredible kindness and generosity.

You're on this noble caregiving journey, and I want to remind you that your well-being deserves the spotlight. Think of it as giving yourself a little TLC to honor your spirit and boost your energy levels. After all, serving others is incredible, but doing it from a place of abundance feels even better than saving the day on an empty tank.

So, let's make a pact to prioritize your well-being. You've got this, and I'm here cheering you on every step of the way! It's time to embrace the superhero within you and let self-care be your cape!

IMPORTANCE OF SELF-CARE FOR CAREGIVERS

It's time to have a heart-to-heart about the twists and turns of dementia caregiving. It's like a roller-coaster, right? And here's the real deal—getting caught up in the whirlwind without realizing the toll it might take on you is easy. We get it; it's no walk in the park, and sometimes, you might feel like you're running on empty. Can you relate? Feeling tired, a bit low, or constantly on edge? You're not alone in this struggle.

But remember, "Only when we first help ourselves can we effectively help others. Caring for yourself is one of the most important —and one of the most often forgotten—things you can do as a caregiver" (*Taking care of you: Self-care for family caregivers*, 2023, para. 1).

How do you know when it's time to prioritize yourself? It's essential to recognize the warning signs. Picture this: trouble falling asleep, consistent low energy levels, and a lingering feeling of persistent sadness. Or maybe you're noticing a shift in your eating habits—either seeking comfort in too much food or losing your appetite altogether. These could be subtle signals that your well-being is taking a hit.

Check in with your emotions. Are irritability and anxiety becoming frequent companions? Feeling overwhelmed by the present or anxious about the future? These emotional shifts might tell you to pause and focus on your needs.

Physical cues are crucial, too. Frequent headaches, muscle tension, or unexplained aches and pains could be your body's way of signaling stress. Your immune system might be hit, making you more susceptible to catching colds or facing other health issues.

Now, let's dive into the mental game. Are concentration and decision-making becoming a challenge? Memory lapses and an overall sense of mental fatigue might be sneaking in. These cognitive signs can impact your ability to navigate caregiving challenges.

Don't forget the social side. If you're withdrawing from friends and family, skipping social gatherings, or feeling isolated, it's time to take notice. Your social connections are like a lifeline, and any change in your social behavior could signal a need for self-care.

In daily interactions, are you finding your patience wearing thin, getting easily frustrated, or feeling hopeless? These emotional responses are like red flags that your stress levels might be hitting a critical point.

Lastly, let's talk about sleep. Any disruptions in your sleep routine —difficulty falling asleep, frequent wake-ups, or restless nights— could be signs that your body and mind need a bit more TLC.

By tuning into these physical and emotional signs, you're arming yourself with the awareness to take proactive steps toward self-care. Remember, recognizing these cues is not a sign of weakness; it's a testament to your strength and self-awareness. Taking care of yourself isn't just important; it's the cornerstone for providing top-notch care to your loved one. You've got this!

COMBATING STRESS AND BURNOUT

Envision stress as a constant, nagging hum in your ears and burnout as the sudden crash against a formidable brick wall. Both are intrusive companions on your caregiving path and learning to recognize their signs is your strategy for steering clear of peril.

Stress is like your body's natural alarm system responding to a demanding situation. It's the wear and tear on your body and mind as you navigate the challenges of caregiving.

But here's the catch–if you let stress run wild, it can wreak havoc on your physical, emotional, and mental well-being. Your body goes into overdrive, releasing stress hormones that, over time, will lead to health issues. Picture it like running a marathon without a water break—it takes a toll.

Symptoms of Stress

Physical Signs

- Headaches or migraines
- Muscle tension and pain
- Digestive issues
- Frequent illnesses due to a weakened immune system

Emotional Signs

- Increased irritability
- Anxiety or constant worry
- Mood swings
- Feelings of helplessness

Cognitive Signs

- Difficulty concentrating
- Memory lapses
- Racing thoughts
- Decision-making challenges

Behavioral Signs

- Changes in eating habits (overeating or loss of appetite)
- Sleep disturbances.
- Social withdrawal
- Increased use of substances (alcohol, caffeine, etc.)

What Is Burnout?

Burnout—it's more than just feeling tired. Burnout is like a storm brewing on the horizon, gradually wearing you down. You're left feeling empty when you've poured so much into caregiving.

When your energy dwindles, your enthusiasm fades, and suddenly, caregiving feels like an impossible task. It's a major roadblock that can seriously impact your well-being and ability to give the best care possible.

Signs of Burnout

Physical Exhaustion

- Chronic fatigue
- Insomnia or disturbed sleep
- Recurrent illnesses

Emotional Detachment

- Feeling emotionally drained
- Loss of empathy
- A sense of hopelessness

Reduced Performance

- Decreased productivity.
- Difficulty concentrating
- Increased mistakes or errors

Interpersonal Issues

- Strained relationships
- Social withdrawal
- Increased conflicts

PRACTICAL SELF-CARE STRATEGIES

Practical self-care is about creating habits that prioritize your well-being. You've got the power to weave self-care into life if you break into small steps. Keep it simple, real, and most importantly, take care of yourself.

- Take mini breaks.
- Schedule "me time."
- Delegate tasks.
- Simplify your space.
- Break tasks up.
- Establish a sleep routine.
- Learn to say no.

CREATING A SELF-CARE PLAN

Creating a self-care plan is like crafting a roadmap for your well-being.

Reflect on Your Needs

- Take a moment to reflect on what makes you feel happy, relaxed, and energized.
- Identify specific areas in your life where you could use more care.

List Your Go-To Activities

- Jot down activities that bring you joy and relaxation.
- Include both big and small things that make you feel good.

Prioritize Your Well-Being

- Identify self-care activities that are non-negotiable for your overall well-being.
- Make a list of top priorities that you commit to regularly.

Schedule Self-Care Time

- Block out dedicated time in your calendar for self-care.
- Treat this time as sacred—just like any other important commitment.

Be Realistic and Flexible

- Set realistic expectations for yourself.
- Be flexible and adjust your plan as needed.

Include Social Connections

- List ways to connect with friends, family, or support groups.
- Prioritize social activities that uplift and rejuvenate you.

Plan for Stressful Times

- Identify self-care strategies specifically for challenging moments.
- Have a plan in place for when stress levels are high.

Mix It Up

- Keep your plan diverse with a mix of activities.
- Rotate through different self-care options to keep things fresh.

Seek Professional Support

- Consider incorporating professional support into your plan.
- Explore counseling, therapy, and other resources that enhance your well-being.

Regularly Review and Adjust

- Schedule regular check-ins with your self-care plan.
- Adjust activities or priorities based on what's working or changing in your life.

Feel free to tweak and adjust as life unfolds. Most importantly, you can shape a plan that best supports you on this caregiving journey.

So, take that first step and create a plan that puts your well-being front and center. You deserve it!

SELF-CARE AND YOUR LOVED ONE

By making self-care a shared adventure, you're not just looking after yourself but building moments of joy and connection that become bright spots in your caregiving story. It's a celebration of shared experiences, teamwork, and the everlasting power of love.

Simple Pleasures You Both Love

- Think of activities that bring smiles to both your faces.
- Think of things like dancing to old tunes, sharing a warm tea, or wandering through a nearby park.

  o These shared experiences add magic to your relationship.

Mindful Chill Time

- Have you ever tried stretching or taking deep breaths together?

  o It's like hitting the pause button on life's chaos and savoring the present moment.
  o It's about finding tranquility together and becoming a more relaxed team.

Let's Get Crafty

- Grab some paint, paper, or any crafty supplies, and unleash your creativity side by side.

○ It's not about perfection; it's about the laughter, mess, and memories you create together.

Spa Vibes at Home

- Transform ordinary days into spa-like retreats within the comfort of your home.

○ Picture soothing baths, gentle massages, or a bit of pampering together.
○ It's not just about self-care; it's about doubling the relaxation and joy.

Nature Date

- Try gardening together, basking in the sunlight, or feeling the breeze against your faces.

○ Nature becomes your playground, offering moments of serenity and shared adventures beyond the everyday.

High-Five for Achievements

- Celebrate every victory, big or small.

○ Completing a puzzle, cooking a meal, or reaching a personal goal are all worth cheering for.

GOAL SETTING FOR CAREGIVERS

Caring for someone with dementia can make taking care of yourself feel like solving a puzzle with extra pieces. It's not always easy to prioritize self-care, but a helpful strategy called SMART goals can make a big difference, especially in dementia caregiving. Let's break it down together.

Specific

Let's get specific about your self-care routine in caregiving. Think about what activities make you feel good and relaxed. It could be spending 20-30 minutes each day listening to soothing music, walking with your loved one, doing some gentle exercises, or just taking a few moments to read quietly.

Measurable

Keep a close eye on your self-care routine and its impact. Use a calendar or an app to monitor how these moments influence your mood, energy levels, and stress in the caregiving journey.

Attainable

Make sure your self-care goals align with the demands of dementia caregiving. Begin with manageable steps, and gradually increase the frequency and duration of your self-care activities, considering the unique challenges of your caregiving role.

Relevant

Select self-care activities that are meaningful and applicable to your role as a dementia caregiver. Avoid activities that may add unnecessary stress and instead focus on what brings comfort and joy.

Time-Based

Give your self-care goals a time frame that accommodates the responsibilities of dementia caregiving. This keeps you focused and motivated and allows for regular evaluations and adjustments.

Regular self-assessment becomes crucial in the realm of dementia caregiving. Consider setting a weekly reminder to check in with yourself, reflect on your caregiving journey, and adapt your self-care goals accordingly.

SMART goals are your tailored guide to crafting an effective self-care routine while caring for a loved one with dementia. Specific, Measurable, Attainable, Relevant, and Time-based—these principles help you set practical goals and keep a vigilant eye on your progress, ensuring a more balanced and fulfilling caregiving life. You've got this, and your well-being matters every step of the way!

SEEKING AND USING SUPPORT NETWORKS

Navigating the challenges of caring for a loved one with dementia is no small feat, and it's okay to seek and embrace support from others.

Family and Friends

Your inner circle—the folks who know you and your loved one like the back of their hand—can be your anchor in stormy seas. Whether it's a heartfelt chat, lending a hand, or simply sharing a laugh, family and friends are priceless treasures. Take the reins and reach out through any means available, whether a phone call, email, text, or a quick message on social media. And hey, don't be shy about spelling out your needs. Maybe you could use a hand with groceries from a family member or a friend to spend quality time with your loved one. Open up about your feelings, seek guidance, and let your support network be the sturdy pillars that lift you.

Community Resources

Do you know many local groups and organizations that help caregivers like you and your loved one? They've got all sorts of services, from giving you a break with respite care to lending a hand with home health tasks. Need a lift to appointments or help with meals? They've got you covered! How do you find them? Start by checking out your Area Agency on Aging, local senior center, hospital, or faith community. And hey, don't forget about the handy online tools like the Eldercare Locator or Alzheimer's and Dementia Caregiver Center—they can also point you in the right direction. So why wait? Reach out and tap into these community resources—they're there to give you the support you need right when needed.

Online Forums

Hey, have you ever thought about diving into online forums for caregivers? They're like treasure troves of shared stories, advice, and support from folks who are right there in the trenches with you. Plus, you can hang out there anonymously, and it's super convenient. There are many places to check out, like CaringBridge, Memory People, Caring for Elderly Parents, Working Daughter, or Caregivers Connect. They're like little corners of the internet where caregivers gather to swap tips and lend a listening ear. And don't forget about social media— Facebook and Twitter can be gold mines, too. Search for keywords related to your caregiving situation, and you'll find a whole world of supportive communities waiting to welcome you with open arms. Trust me, you're not alone in this journey—there are plenty of folks out there ready to walk alongside you every step of the way.

Asking for Help

You know, asking for help might be one of the bravest things you can do on this caregiving adventure. It's not about admitting defeat but showing your strength and connecting with others who want to lend a hand. Think of it like forming your own superhero team—because, let's face it, being a caregiver is pretty darn heroic, and heroes deserve backup. So, don't be afraid to reach out when you need it. You've got a whole squad of support waiting to join forces.

Here are some detailed tips to guide you:

Be Specific

- When asking for assistance, provide precise details.

  ○ Specify tasks (picking up groceries, helping with household chores, etc.).

Share Your Feelings

- Openly express how you're doing.

  ○ If you feel overwhelmed or need a break, communicate these feelings to your support network.

- Honest communication fosters understanding and empathy.

Express Gratitude

- Acknowledge and appreciate the help you receive.

  ○ A simple thank-you goes a long way in reinforcing the support you receive from others.

Create a Network

- Recognize the strengths of different individuals in your network.
- Diversifying your support network ensures a well-rounded caregiving support system.

Prioritize Self-Care

- Understand that asking for help is not just about fulfilling your caregiving duties; it's also about taking care of yourself.
- Prioritize self-care and communicate your need for breaks to ensure your well-being.

CAREGIVING TIPS FOR BALANCING TIME WITH FAMILY, FRIENDS, AND YOURSELF

The road of caring for someone with dementia is a challenging one, especially when you are also balancing all the demands of your everyday life, especially if you are raising kids. In the United States, around 25% of households are grappling with caregiving challenges, which are expected to rise as the baby boomers age (Shapiro, 2018).

Whether you are caring for a family member, a dear friend, or someone else, achieving the right balance is essential. It is important to consider having multiple caregivers, as it allows a rotation schedule for responsibilities. When you can rotate, it will enable your loved one to receive continuous support while giving you the time to take a much-needed break.

You must have a good grasp of your loved one's capabilities, daily needs, and preferred activities before you devise your loved one's schedule. It is also important to properly assess if they will need constant supervision.

Recognizing that formal training may not be in your caregiving toolkit is essential. As a family caregiver, you are likely navigating financial matters, managing medical appointments, and providing hands-on care, which is a full-time job. On top of any other responsibilities you might have.

Be Realistic About Your Limitations

Acknowledging what you can realistically handle is a cornerstone of effective caregiving. Recognize that setting boundaries is healthy and essential for sustaining your caregiving journey.

Example

- If you feel stretched thin, consider creating a list of tasks with which others in your support network can assist. Delegating responsibilities lightens the load and allows you to focus on critical aspects of care.

Cooperate With Others

You are not a lone superhero; you are part of a team. Seek help and foster cooperation with others in your support network. Building a collaborative caregiving network is invaluable, whether it is family members, friends, or hired assistance.

Example

- Establish regular check-ins or family meetings to discuss the caregiving plan. This creates a shared understanding and allows everyone to contribute strengths to the caregiving journey.

Take Daily Breaks for Self-Care

Self-care is not a luxury; it is a necessity. Incorporate daily breaks into your routine to recharge mentally and emotionally. These moments are like fuel for the caregiving engine.

Example

- Designate specific times during the day for short breaks. It could be a morning meditation session, an afternoon walk, or a few minutes of quiet decompression time.

Schedule Vacations to Recharge

Caregiving is demanding, and you deserve periodic respites. Plan vacations, brief getaways, or extended breaks to recharge and return to caregiving with a fresh perspective.

Example

- Plan a week-long break by coordinating with other caregivers or support services. It is not just a break for you but an opportunity for your loved one to experience different caregiving styles.

Denial about your loved one's illness is a common coping mechanism, but facing the reality is crucial for effective coping and overall well-being. It is a journey filled with challenges, but remember, you are not alone.

Do not hesitate to ask for and accept help. Your well-being is a priority and the foundation for sustained caregiving excellence. You are navigating this with strength and grace; your dedication is commendable!

BALANCING CAREGIVING AND YOUR PERSONAL LIFE

Managing the whirlwind of caregiving duties while tending to your personal life is like walking a tightrope. But fear not, my friend, because mastering this balancing act is the key to keeping everything in harmony.

Think of it as nurturing a garden. Just like forgetting to water the plants can stunt their growth, neglecting your own well-being can hinder your ability to provide the care your loved one needs. Your well-being isn't just a nice-to-have—it's essential for your superhero role as a caregiver. You can give your best care when you're physically, emotionally, and mentally in a good place.

Finding this balance isn't a one-time thing—it's an ongoing journey, like driving a car and knowing when to pull over for gas. Your well-being is the fuel that keeps you going. So, when life throws curveballs, don't forget to check your emotional tank, and refuel as needed.

Imagine sailing through stormy seas as the captain of your ship. Being adaptable and willing to change course when necessary, guides you to calmer waters. But beware: neglecting this balance can affect your health, like a phone battery draining too quickly without a recharge.

Remember, taking care of yourself isn't selfish—it's like securing your own oxygen mask before assisting others on a plane. Your loved one depends on you, and by prioritizing your well-being, you're helping yourself and enhancing the care you provide.

Reach out to your support network—whether it's friends, family, or fellow caregivers. Sharing your journey, celebrating the victories, and seeking guidance can offer comfort and valuable insights.

You've got the strength to tackle the challenges ahead. By finding this delicate balance, you're not just sustaining yourself—you're ensuring that you can continue to be the compassionate rock for your loved one with dementia. So, take a moment to breathe, don't hesitate to ask for help when needed, and keep nurturing your personal life and role as a caring caregiver. You've got this!

CLOSING THOUGHTS

Let's recap what we've covered in this chapter—it's been quite the journey! You've delved into the importance of caring for your loved one and caring for yourself along the way. Together, we've explored some practical strategies to tackle stress, manage those overwhelming emotions, and seek the support you need. But hold onto your hat because our journey isn't over yet!

Now, let's talk about planning—crucial for your and your loved one's future. Planning ahead can be your secret weapon, helping you avoid unexpected crises, ease uncertainties, and safeguard your rights and interests.

In the next chapter, "All About Planning," we'll explore the nitty-gritty of financial and legal planning tailored to dementia care. We'll cover everything from budgeting and insurance to assistance programs, wills, trusts, and power of attorney. By the time you've finished reading, you'll have a solid grasp on how to create the best care plan for you and your loved one.

BE A SUPERHERO WITH YOUR REVIEW!

UNLOCK THE MAGIC OF HELPING OTHERS

Doing good for others is like a boomerang; it always comes back to you! - Imagine that said by a wise old owl.

Did you know doing good for others without expecting a return makes people happiest? They smile, laugh, and make more friends. Let's be those happy people together, okay?

Now, I've got a super special favor to ask you...

Would you be a secret hero for someone you've never met without getting credit? With your invisible cape, you could anonymously brighten their day.

Who is this mystery person, you wonder? Well, they're a bit like you of yesterday—maybe a little unsure, wanting to make a big splash in the world and looking for a guiding light.

Our mission is to make dementia care as simple and comforting as pie with "The Dementia Caregiver's Toolkit." Every part of this book is crafted to achieve this goal, aiming to reach everyone!

Your superhero cape is needed! Many pick books by their covers and reviews. I'm asking you to be a hero for a fellow dementia caregiver, a kindred spirit you might never meet but who shares our mission.

Please help the caregiver of someone with dementia by leaving this book a review.

Your gift costs no money and takes less than 60 seconds to make it real. Still, it can change a fellow dementia caregiver's life forever. Your review could be the reason...

- ...another family feels a little less alone in their journey.
- ...another caregiver finds the strength to face the day.
- ...someone out there gets a helping hand when they need it most.
- ...a light bulb goes on, and things start to make sense for someone struggling.
- ...a dream of making caregiving a bit easier comes true.

To get that 'feel good' sensation and truly make a difference for this individual, all you have to do is... and it takes less than 60 seconds... leave a review.

Just zap the QR code below with your phone to leave your review:

SCAN ME

If the thought of doing this secret good deed makes you feel warm and fuzzy, then you're my kind of superhero. Welcome to the team. You're one of the good ones.

I can't wait to show you how to make the caregiving journey less scary, more manageable, and full of love in ways you never imagined. The tips coming up are going to be awesome.

Thank you. Your contribution is genuinely super heroic - and it means everything to me. So, are you ready to turn the page and continue this journey?

- Your biggest cheerleader, Tina E. Bradley

PS - Every act of kindness plants a seed of joy. Could this book help another caregiver? Sharing it could light up their path. Let's spread happiness together - share the book and brighten someone's journey!

5

ALL ABOUT PLANNING

The only way to get through life is to laugh your way through it. You either have to laugh or cry. I prefer to laugh. Crying gives me a headache.

— MARJORIE PAY HINCKLEY (HINCKLEY, 1999, P. 107)

This quote captures the spirit of this chapter, which is about planning for the financial and legal aspects of dementia care. While this may seem daunting and stressful, it is also an opportunity to find some relief in the middle of uncertainty. Planning can help you avoid pitfalls and prepare for the future with confidence and peace of mind. It can also allow you to focus more on caregiving's positive moments and joys rather than worrying about the costs and complications.

BUDGETING FOR DEMENTIA CARE COSTS

Navigating the financial side of dementia care requires a thoughtful and strategic approach.

"The average monthly cost of memory care in the United States is $6,935, according to 2021 NIC statistics. This is more expensive than typical assisted living (about $4,500/month) but less than a private room in a nursing home ($9,034)" (Pedersen, 2023, para. 4).

Assess Finances

- Start by understanding your current financial situation. Identify your income sources, savings, and any existing insurance.

Estimate Dementia Care Costs

- Research and estimate all potential costs associated with dementia care, including medical expenses, medications, in-home care, or facility costs.

Create a Monthly Budget

- Develop a monthly budget that outlines your income and all anticipated expenses.

Explore Assistance Programs

- Check out government assistance programs like Medicaid or Veterans Affairs for potential financial support.

Check Long-Term Care Insurance

- If you don't have it, consider long-term care insurance. It can cover in-home care, assisted living, or nursing home costs.

Consult a Financial Advisor

- Get advice from a financial advisor with expertise in healthcare and long-term care planning.

Explore Community Resources

- Look into local organizations or support groups that might offer assistance or cost-saving information.

Prioritize Essential Expenses

- Ensure your budget prioritizes crucial needs.

Plan for Future Costs

- Anticipate potential future costs as dementia progresses, adjusting your budget accordingly.

Review and Adjust

- Regularly review and adjust your budget as circumstances change, ensuring it stays aligned with your needs.

Explore Alternative Care Options

- Investigate cost-effective alternatives such as community-based programs, adult day care, or respite care.

Consider Legal and Estate Planning

- Consult legal and financial professionals for estate planning to protect assets and ease financial transitions.

Budgeting thoughtfully ensures financial stability and the best care for your loved one. By regularly reviewing and adjusting your budget, you're actively contributing to effective financial planning.

Practical Tips for Budgeting

Coping with the unique financial demands of dementia care requires thoughtful budgeting.

Shared Living Arrangements

- Explore shared living options, where individuals with dementia share accommodations.

  ○ While more cost-effective, it may lack the security of a dedicated memory care unit.

Review Income and Assets

- Assess the income sources and assets of both you and your loved one.

 ○ Understand the available funds from pensions, Social Security, investments, savings, property, or insurance.

Research Dementia Care Options

- Compare different care types (memory care, home care, adult day care) and their costs.
- Inquire about services, amenities, and potential financial assistance.

 ○ Check for discounts or subsidies.

Create a Monthly Budget

- List all income and expenses related to your loved one's dementia care, including fees, wages, medical bills, legal fees, home modifications, transportation, or respite care.
- Balance the budget, allowing for unexpected costs and emergencies.

Monitor and Update Regularly

- Track your income and expenses, comparing them with the budget.
- Adjust as needed and review the budget every 6 months or with significant changes in your loved one's condition.

Taking care to budget thoughtfully ensures financial stability and the best care for your loved one. You're actively contributing to effective financial planning by regularly reviewing and adjusting your budget.

Government-Funded Programs: Financial Assistance Programs for Dementia Caregivers

Government-funded programs are designed to provide you with financial assistance and support. Exploring these programs can make a big difference in dealing with care costs, offering you and your loved one support and resources.

Medicaid: Essential Medical Coverage

- Medicaid provides coverage for medical and long-term care services.
- Services include hospital visits, doctor appointments, prescription medications, and nursing home care.
- Eligibility is based on income and varies by state.

Veterans Affairs (VA) Benefits: Honoring Service

- The VA offers Aid and Attendance (A&A) and Housebound benefits.
- A&A provides extra funds for those needing assistance with daily activities.
- Housebound benefits support those with permanent disability leading to confinement at home.

Area Agencies on Aging (AAA): Localized Assistance

- AAAs assist older adults and caregivers with information, resources, and direct services.
- Support programs, counseling services, and local resource navigation are common offerings.

Supplemental Security Income (SSI): Financial Aid for Low-Income Individuals

- SSI provides financial assistance to elderly, blind, or disabled individuals with limited income and resources.
- Eligibility is tied to the income and assets of the caregiver and the person receiving care.

National Family Caregiver Support Program (NFCSP): Tailored Assistance

- NFCSP offers information, assistance, counseling, support groups, and respite care for family caregivers.
- Services may vary by location, focusing on addressing caregivers' unique needs.

Social Security Disability Insurance (SSDI): Aid for Disabled Individuals

- SSDI provides financial assistance to individuals with disabilities, including those with early-onset dementia.
- Monthly payments and auxiliary benefits may be available.
- Eligibility criteria include work history and severity of disability.

Community Development Block Grants (CDBG): Localized Support

- CDBG funds support local communities with various development needs.
- Some communities allocate funds to assist caregivers through programs like home modifications, transportation aid, or caregiver training.

- Explore available CDBG-funded initiatives through local government channels.

Setting Up an Emergency Fund

Being prepared for unexpected challenges is crucial for caregivers. One way to build financial resilience is by setting up an emergency fund. This fund provides a safety net for unforeseen expenses, offering peace of mind during the caregiving journey.

An emergency fund is a savings account specifically dedicated to covering unexpected expenses. It provides a financial cushion, allowing you to handle unforeseen circumstances without compromising your budget.

Steps to Establish Your Emergency Fund

- Start small.
- Calculate how much you can comfortably set aside each month.
- Explore high-interest savings accounts.
- Resist the urge to dip into your emergency fund for non-emergencies.
- Regularly review and adjust.

As a caregiver, this fund allows you to focus on your loved one's well-being without added financial stress. You're creating a financial safety net that provides security during unexpected challenges.

NAVIGATING INSURANCE AND ASSISTANCE PROGRAMS

When dealing with the complexities of caregiving, especially as you prepare for the end of life, it is also crucial to tackle insurance and assistance programs directly.

Check Your Insurance Policies:

- Understand what's included and any limitations related to end-of-life care.

Explore Government Assistance:

- Look into government assistance programs like Medicaid or Veterans Affairs benefits.

Consult Social Workers or Care Coordinators:

- Seek guidance from social workers or care coordinators who can help you understand available programs, assist with applications, and advocate for your loved one's needs.

Tap into Community Resources:

- Explore local community resources and nonprofit organizations that may offer financial aid, volunteer services, or emotional support during the challenging time of end-of-life care.

Be an Advocate:

- Stand up for your loved one's needs.

Plan for Funeral Expenses:

- Consider pre-arranged funeral plans or burial insurance to ease the financial burden on the family after your loved one passes.

UNDERSTANDING GOVERNMENT BENEFITS

Looking after a family member with dementia comes with its unique set of challenges and one big hurdle is the financial strain it can put on you and your family. The expenses for medical care, medications, and long-term care services can pile up, squeezing your budget. But here's the silver lining–there are government programs out there that can lend a hand, helping to cover some of these costs and ease your financial load. Now, I get it. Figuring out the eligibility criteria and application process can feel like navigating a maze. But worry not! I'm here to give you straightforward information on the various government benefits that could be a game-changer for you and your loved ones.

Medicare

Medicare is an insurance plan for people aged 65 and older, those with disabilities, and those with certain chronic conditions.

Each part of Medicare addresses specific healthcare expenses, providing a comprehensive approach to coverage.

Part A (Hospital Insurance)

- Inpatient hospital stays,
- Skilled nursing facility care,
- Hospice care.

THE DEMENTIA CAREGIVER'S TOOLKIT | 137

Part B (Medical Insurance)

- Outpatient care,
- Doctor visits,
- Preventive services,
- Some home health care (not covered by Part A),
- Requires a monthly premium.

Part C (Medicare Advantage)

- Combines coverage from Part A, Part B, and sometimes Part D,
- May include additional benefits beyond the Original Medicare,
- These plans often include additional benefits and may have different costs.

Part D (Prescription Drug Coverage)

- Offers prescription drug coverage,
- Can be added to Original Medicare or included in some Medicare Advantage plans,
- Requires a separate premium.

To be eligible for Medicare, you or your loved one must be a US citizen or legally living in the US for at least five years.

Also, you need to meet one of the following criteria:

- Be 65 or older and eligible for Social Security or Railroad Retirement benefits.
- Be under 65 and have a disability that has lasted or is expected to last at least 24 months.

- Have end-stage renal disease (permanent kidney failure that requires dialysis or a transplant).
- Have amyotrophic lateral sclerosis (ALS, also known as Lou Gehrig's disease).

To apply for Medicare, you can do one of the following:

- Visit the Social Security website at ssa.gov or call 1-800-772-1213.
- Visit the Railroad Retirement Board website at rrb.gov or call 1-877-772-5772.

Suppose you already have Social Security or Railroad Retirement benefits. In that case, you will automatically qualify for Medicare Part A and B when you turn 65 or become disabled. You'll get your Medicare card by mail about three months before you become eligible. You can decline Part B if you do not want it, but you may have to pay a penalty if you enroll later.

Medigap

Medigap is supplemental insurance that covers costs not paid by Medicare. Private insurance companies sell standardized plans. Each Medigap plan provides different levels of coverage, allowing individuals to choose a plan that best fits their healthcare needs and preferences.

Plan A

- Basic coverage, including coinsurance for hospital costs and 365 additional days of hospital care after Medicare benefits end.

Plan B

- Covers everything in Plan A, plus Part A deductible and Part B coinsurance.

Plan C

- Includes coverage from Plan B and for skilled nursing facility coinsurance, Part B deductible, and limited foreign travel emergency coverage.

Plan D

- Covers everything in Plan C, excluding the Part B deductible.

Plan F

- The most comprehensive coverage includes all Plan D benefits and full coverage for the Part B deductible.

Plan G

- Similar to Plan F, but does not cover the Part B deductible.

Plan K

- Offers partial coverage for certain expenses, such as hospital and preventive care.

Plan L

- Provides another level of partial coverage for hospital and preventive care, with lower out-of-pocket limits.

Plan M

- Covers similar expenses as Plan D but with lower cost-sharing requirements.

Plan N

- Similar to Plan D, with added coverage for Part B coinsurance and some co-payments.

Medigap can be a valuable option for dementia caregivers and their loved ones who want to reduce their medical expenses and have more predictable costs. It's essential to carefully review and understand the specific coverage limitations of each Medigap plan to ensure you have the necessary coverage for your healthcare needs.

Here's a list of what is generally not covered by Medigap plans:

Prescription Drugs

- Medigap plans do not cover prescription drug costs. You must enroll in a separate Medicare Part D plan for prescription drug coverage.

Long-Term Care

- Costs related to long-term care in a nursing home or assisted living facility are not covered.

Dental Care

- Routine dental care, including check-ups, cleanings, and most dental procedures, is not covered by Medigap.

Vision Care

- Medigap plans generally do not cover eye exams, glasses, and contact lenses.

Hearing Aids

- Costs associated with hearing aids and hearing exams are not covered.

Eyeglasses

- The cost of eyeglasses is not covered by Medigap insurance.

Private Nursing

- Medigap plans do not cover private-duty nursing services.

Overseas Care (Except for Plan C and Plan F)

- Medigap plans typically do not cover healthcare services obtained outside of the United States, except for Plan C and Plan F.

To qualify for Medigap, you or your loved one must have Medicare Part A and B and be within one of the following enrollment periods:

- The enrollment period is 6 months, starting at age 65 or when you enroll in Part B, whichever is later. During this period, you have a guaranteed right to buy any Medigap plan available in your state, regardless of your health status or history.
- The open enrollment period, from October 15 to December 7, is when you can switch or drop your Medigap plan. However, you may have to go through medical underwriting and pay higher premiums or be denied coverage based on your health condition.
- The special enrollment period is triggered by certain life events, such as losing your employer-sponsored coverage, moving out of your plan's service area, or your plan going bankrupt. Depending on the circumstances, you may have a guaranteed right to buy a Medigap plan during this period.

To apply for Medigap, you can do one of the following:

- Compare and shop for Medigap plans online at medicare.gov or call 1-800-MEDICARE.
- For free counseling and assistance, contact your state health insurance assistance program (SHIP) at shiptacenter.org or call 1-877-839-2675.

You can contact the insurance company directly or work with a licensed agent or broker to get insurance.

Medicaid

Medicaid is a collaborative federal and state program to provide health coverage for low-income elderly, disabled, and chronically ill individuals.

Here's a breakdown of what Medicaid can cover:

Health Coverage for Targeted Groups

- Specifically, it caters to low-income elderly, disabled, and chronically ill individuals.

Long-Term Care Services for Dementia

- Medicaid can assist in covering various long-term care services for individuals with dementia.

  - Nursing home care
  - Assisted Living
  - Home and community-based services
  - Personal care

Limitations on Long-Term Care Services

- It's important to note that Medicaid does not cover all long-term care services. The availability and eligibility for these services may vary by state.

Eligibility Criteria

- To qualify for Medicaid, individuals must meet specific eligibility criteria, including:

  - Income and asset limits
  - Functional and medical criteria

Varied Income and Asset Limits

- The income and asset limits for Medicaid eligibility are contingent on factors such as:

  ○ State regulations
  ○ Household size
  ○ Type of coverage sought

Comprehensive Assessment for Abilities and Needs

- Medicaid eligibility is determined through a comprehensive assessment, considering both physical and mental capabilities.

  ○ This assessment helps tailor the coverage to the individual's specific needs.

Understanding Medicaid's coverage and eligibility criteria is essential for those seeking assistance with long-term care services for individuals with dementia. Remember that the details may vary by state, so it's advisable to check the specific requirements in your location (Garfield, 2015).

To apply for Medicaid, you can do one of the following:

- Visit the Medicaid website at medicaid.gov or call 1-877-267-2323.
- Visit the HealthCare.gov website at healthcare.gov or call 1-800-318-2596.

Contact your state Medicaid agency or local social services office for more information and assistance.

SSDI and SSI

SSDI and SSI are federal programs that provide cash benefits to disabled individuals who cannot work. SSDI is based on your work history and contributions to Social Security. In contrast, SSI is based on your financial need and other factors. Both programs can help you pay for your living expenses and qualify for other benefits, such as Medicare and Medicaid.

SSDI and SSI Criteria

- Individuals with disabilities who cannot work at the level of substantial gainful activity (SGA) defined by Social Security.
- Have a disability that has lasted or is expected to last at least 12 months or result in death.
- Have a disability that meets or exceeds the criteria of Social Security's Listing of Impairments, which includes dementia and related disorders.
- For SSDI, have enough work credits based on your age and earnings.
- For SSI, they have limited income and resources below a certain threshold.

To apply for SSDI or SSI, you can do one of the following:

- Visit the Social Security website at ssa.gov or call 1-800-772-1213.
- Visit your local Social Security office or schedule an appointment.

Suppose you are diagnosed with early-onset Alzheimer's disease or another form of dementia. In that case, you may qualify for the

Compassionate Allowances program, which can expedite your application process and grant you benefits faster. You can find more information about this program at https://www.ssa.gov/compassionateallowances/.

Checklist of Documents Needed

When applying for government benefits, you will need to provide various documents and information, such as:

- Social Security card or number.
- Birth certificate or other proof of age.
- US passport or other proof of citizenship or legal residency.
- W-2 forms, tax returns, pay stubs, or other proof of income.
- Bank statements, property deeds, vehicle titles, or other proof of assets.
- Medical records, doctor reports, test results, or other proof of disability and medical condition.
- A letter from your doctor stating your diagnosis, symptoms, treatment, and prognosis.
- A letter from your employer or former employer stating your work history, duties, and earnings.
- A completed application form for the benefits program you are applying for.

You should keep copies of all the documents you submit and track the status of your application. You should also be prepared to answer questions and provide more information if the agency requests it. If your application is denied, you can appeal the decision and request a hearing.

LEGAL PREPAREDNESS: WILLS AND ADVANCED DIRECTIVES

One of the important aspects of planning for the future after a dementia diagnosis is to make sure that your loved one's legal affairs are in order. This means having a will and advanced directives, which can serve them and your family in several ways.

Ensuring your loved one's wishes are respected and their legacy is thoughtfully managed involves key legal documents.

Will

- Expresses how your loved one desires the distribution of their money, property, and possessions after their passing.
- Ensures their wishes are honored, providing care for their loved ones.
- Helps prevent family disputes and complications, reducing potential taxes and fees.

Advanced Directives

- Empower your loved one to articulate preferences and health and social care decisions in advance.
- Ensures their care aligns with their values and beliefs.
- Provides guidance for family and healthcare professionals, avoiding uncertainty.
- Eases the burden on family members, reducing stress and potential conflicts during challenging times.

Having these essential legal documents in place not only safeguards your loved one's wishes but also brings a sense of security and understanding to everyone involved.

Creating Legal Documents Help

Understand Your Loved One's Situation

- Reflect on your loved one's current needs and situation.
- Consider their preferences for the future, considering financial, personal, and medical aspects.
- Think about how circumstances may change over time.

Choose Trusted Individuals

- Select people your loved one trusts to act on their behalf.
- This person, known as the attorney (for a lasting power of attorney) or executor (for a will), will carry out their wishes when they cannot.

  ○ Ensure they are trustworthy and capable of fulfilling this role.

Complete Relevant Forms

- Fill out the necessary forms for creating a will and advanced directives. These can be found online or obtained from a solicitor.
- Ensure the forms are clear, accurate, and reflect your loved one's wishes.
- Sign them in the presence of two independent witnesses who are not beneficiaries or attorneys.

Register and Safeguard Documents

- If creating a lasting power of attorney (LPA), register it with the Office of the Public Guardian (OPG).

- Keep the will and advanced directives secure, like with a solicitor or a trusted friend.
- For accessibility, inform family and healthcare professionals about the location of these documents.

By following these steps, you can make the process of creating legal documents more understandable and ensure that your loved one's wishes are documented and protected compassionately.

Helpful Legal Advice and Support Resources

- The Alzheimer's Association offers a free online tool called Alzheimer's Navigator to help you find local legal services and resources and create a personalized action plan for your caregiving needs.
- The National Academy of Elder Law Attorneys (NAELA) has a directory of attorneys specializing in elder law and disability issues. You can search by location, name, or area of practice to find a qualified lawyer near you.
- The Legal Services Corporation (LSC) is a nonprofit organization that provides civil legal aid to low-income Americans. You can use their online map to find a legal aid program in your state or territory that can help you with legal issues related to dementia care.
- The National Center on Law and Elder Rights (NCLER) provides free legal training, case consultation, and technical assistance to legal and aging network professionals.
- The National Elder Law Foundation (NELF) is a nonprofit organization certifying attorneys as elder law specialists. You can use the search tool on their website to find a certified elder law attorney (CELA) in your area who has demonstrated expertise and experience in elder law issues.

Tips for Discussing Long-Term Care

Choose the Right Time and Setting

- Find a quiet and comfortable environment to have the conversation, ensuring your loved one feels at ease and focused.
- Approaching the topic of long-term care with care and consideration can foster a positive and collaborative discussion, leading to informed decisions that prioritize your loved one's well-being.

Approach With Sensitivity

- Begin the discussion with empathy and sensitivity, acknowledging that it's a delicate topic and expressing your concern for their well-being.

Listen Actively

- Allow your loved one to share their thoughts and concerns. Active listening fosters open communication and helps build trust.

Share Information

- Provide clear and relevant information about long-term care options, including assisted living, nursing homes, and home care. Ensure they understand the available choices.

Involve Them in Decision-Making

- Empower your loved one by involving them in the decision-making process. Ask for their preferences and consider their input in planning for their care.

Discuss Finances

- Address financial considerations openly and transparently. Explore available resources, insurance coverage, and potential costs associated with long-term care.

Include Family Members

- If appropriate, include other family members in the conversation to ensure everyone is on the same page and can provide support.

Highlight the Benefits of Planning Ahead

- Emphasize the benefits of planning for long-term care in advance, such as having more control over decisions and ensuring their preferences are respected.

Explore In-Home Care Options

- Discuss the possibility of in-home care services, if suitable. Many individuals prefer the comfort of their own homes while receiving necessary assistance.

Be Patient and Reassuring

- Recognize that discussing long-term care can be emotional. Be patient, provide reassurance, and offer ongoing support throughout decision-making.

Developing and sustaining positive connections with those who matter—your family, friends, and healthcare professionals is crucial. These relationships offer emotional backing, hands-on help, and expert advice throughout the caregiving journey. They play a vital role in improving the quality of life for your loved one, fostering a sense of connection and value.

CLOSING THOUGHTS

In the upcoming chapter, "Fostering Healthy Relationships," we'll delve into nurturing these connections and overcoming common challenges. As you conclude the chapter, you'll gain valuable knowledge on fostering relationships that support your well-being and that of your loved one.

6

FOSTERING HEALTHY RELATIONSHIPS

"When you are a caregiver, you know that every day you will touch a life or a life will touch yours."

— UNKNOWN (*100 CAREGIVER QUOTES*, 2020, PARA. 59)

This quote speaks volumes to what we've explored in this chapter, touching on the core of strong connections: acceptance, empathy, and kindness. It prompts us to cherish our loved ones with dementia for who they are and the joy they bring into our lives rather than seeking perfection. It also encourages you to treat yourself with the same gentleness, recognizing your capabilities and vulnerabilities as we navigate this path together.

KEEPING PERSONAL RELATIONSHIPS ALIVE

Taking on the role of a caregiver can deeply impact your connections with others, bringing both challenges and opportunities for growth. You may encounter a range of obstacles in maintaining and strengthening these relationships, including:

- Dealing with criticism, expectations, or exclusion from others who do not understand the reality of caregiving.
- Feeling isolated, lonely, or guilty for asking for or accepting help from others.
- Having less time, energy, or resources to socialize or participate in other activities.
- Experiencing changes in the roles, dynamics, or intimacy of your relationship with your loved one.

However, personal relationships serve as crucial support pillars, offering comfort, understanding, and moments of joy in your life.

To ensure these relationships remain vibrant and fulfilling, prioritize them by:

- Communicating openly and honestly with others about your situation, needs, and feelings.
- Asking for and accepting help from others with specific tasks or respite care.
- Finding ways to adapt and enjoy activities and events with your loved one and others.
- Appreciate and express gratitude for those caring about you and your loved one.

STAYING CONNECTED WITH FRIENDS AND FAMILY

Connecting with friends and family is important for your mental and emotional well-being. It helps you feel like you belong and reminds you of your identity. So, make sure to reach out and keep those connections strong!

Schedule Regular Time for Social Activities

- You should plan and set aside some time each week or month for socializing with your friends and family.

  ○ This could be anything from a phone call, a video chat, a coffee date, a movie night, or a group outing.

Accept Help From Others

- Do not hesitate to ask for and accept help from your friends and family, whether with caregiving tasks, household chores, errands, or respite care.

  ○ This can reduce the stress and burden of caregiving and create opportunities for social interaction and support.
  ○ You could also use online platforms or apps to coordinate and communicate with your helpers.

Join a Support Group or Community

- You will find it helpful to join a support group or community of caregivers who share similar experiences and can provide support and advice.

  ○ This can provide a safe and supportive space to express your feelings, exchange information, and receive advice and encouragement.

- You can find support groups online or face-to-face, depending on your preference.

Adapt and Enjoy Activities and Events With Loved One

- Adapt and modify them to suit your caregiving situation and your loved ones' needs and abilities.

    ○ For example, you can celebrate at home, use online platforms, or involve your loved one in the activities.
    ○ This can help you and your loved one to have fun and create positive memories.

DEALING WITH FAMILY DYNAMICS

Helping a family member with dementia can stir up a whirlwind of emotions, and navigating the complexities of family dynamics becomes incredibly important.

Open Communication

- Establishing a supportive dialogue helps each other understand their perspectives.

Active Listening

- Practice active listening when family members share their concerns or opinions.

Acknowledging Emotions

- Acknowledge the feelings of frustration, sadness, or stress that family members may be experiencing.

Understanding Different Roles

- Appreciate that each family member may play a unique role in supporting their loved one.
- Recognize and value the contributions each person brings.

Sharing Responsibilities

- Create a shared support plan that distributes responsibilities among family members.

Family Meetings

- Schedule regular family meetings to discuss support plans, share updates, and address any concerns.

Setting Realistic Expectations

- Understanding limitations helps in preventing unnecessary strain on relationships.

Seeking External Support

- Consider involving a mediator or counselor to facilitate discussions and help navigate challenging family dynamics if necessary.

Respecting Differences

- Respect differing opinions and approaches to supporting a loved one with dementia.

○ Each family member may have ideas about what is best for their loved one.

Celebrating Small Wins

- Celebrate the small victories and milestones in supporting a family member with dementia together.

FACILITATING FAMILY MEETINGS FOR DEMENTIA CAREGIVING

Hosting family meetings is not just about ticking off to-dos—it's creating a magical space where love, laughter, and collaboration reign supreme. It is an act of love, uniting family members in the shared responsibility of caring for a loved one with dementia. By approaching discussions with empathy and openness, you create a collaborative environment where everyone feels valued, heard, and actively involved in the caregiving journey.

Heartfelt Invitation

- Extend a warm and heartfelt invitation to all family members.
- Emphasize the importance of collective support and encourage open communication.
- Ensure everyone feels valued and heard.

Establishing a Safe Space

- Create a safe and non-judgmental space for discussions.
- Emphasize that the goal is to collaborate and share insights, not to assign blame.

○ A safe environment encourages open dialogue.

Setting an Agenda With Empathy

- Prepare a thoughtful agenda that addresses the immediate needs of your loved one.
- Approach topics with empathy, understanding that each family member may have different perspectives and concerns.

Active Listening

- Encourage active listening during the meeting.
- Ensure that each family member has an opportunity to express their thoughts and feelings.

○ Validate their perspectives, fostering a sense of inclusivity.

Understanding Each Member's Role

- Clarify individual roles and responsibilities within the caregiving journey.
- Discuss how each family member can contribute based on their strengths, availability, and skills.

○ Establishing clear roles minimizes misunderstandings.

Sharing Information

- Share relevant information about your loved one's condition, medical updates, and changes in their needs.
- Transparent communication ensures that everyone is well-informed and can actively participate in decision-making.

Problem-Solving Collaboratively

- Approach challenges as a team.
- Brainstorm together and seek collaborative solutions.

  ○ This collective problem-solving approach fosters a sense of unity and shared responsibility.

Addressing Financial Considerations

- Discuss financial aspects openly.
- Address concerns related to the cost of care, potential financial assistance, and the equitable distribution of responsibilities.

  ○ Transparency about financial matters prevents misunderstandings.

Scheduling Regular Check-Ins

- Establish a schedule for regular family meetings.
- Consistent communication allows for updates, adjustments to the care plan, and ongoing collaboration.
- Regular check-ins promote a sense of shared commitment.

Expressing Gratitude

- Acknowledge and express gratitude for each family member's contributions.
- Recognize the unique strengths they bring to the caregiving journey.

CREATING A FAMILY CARE PLAN FOR CAREGIVING

Creating a family care plan is like crafting a roadmap that brings everyone together on the same journey, ensuring harmony and support at every step. It's a way to ensure we're all working together to provide the best care possible.

Heartfelt Reflection

- Begin by reflecting on your loved one's needs, preferences, and your family's unique dynamics.
- Consider everyone's strengths, limitations, and availability.

Open Communication

- Foster an environment of open and honest communication.
- Encourage family members to share their thoughts, concerns, and commitments. Create a safe space where everyone feels heard and valued.

Identify Roles and Responsibilities

- Assign specific roles and responsibilities to each family member based on their abilities and availability.
- Ensure that everyone understands their unique contribution to the caregiving journey.

Shared Decision-Making

- Make decisions collaboratively, considering input from all family members.

- Emphasize the importance of shared decision-making to ensure everyone feels involved and invested in the caregiving process.

Flexible Scheduling

- Acknowledge the unpredictability of caregiving.
- Create a flexible schedule that accommodates the changing needs of your loved one.
- This flexibility allows for adjustments as circumstances evolve.

Financial Considerations

- Discuss and plan for the financial aspects of caregiving.

  ○ Address potential costs, allocate resources, and explore financial assistance options.
  ○ Transparency about financial matters fosters trust and understanding.

Emotional Support Strategies

- Recognize the emotional toll caregiving may have on family members.
- Develop strategies to provide emotional support, such as regular check-ins, shared activities, or access to counseling services.

Emergency Preparedness

- Plan for unexpected situations by outlining emergency protocols.

- Communicate what steps must be taken in case of unforeseen events, ensuring everyone is well-prepared for any scenario.

Regular Family Meetings

- Schedule regular family meetings to discuss updates, care plan adjustments, and emerging challenges.
- These meetings provide a forum for continuous communication and adaptation.

Celebrate Victories Together

- Acknowledge and celebrate the victories, no matter how small.
- Recognize and appreciate the collective effort of the family in providing care and support.

STRENGTHENING BONDS WITH YOUR LOVED ONE

Going through the tough road of dementia can feel like the person you love is slipping away. Memories blur, thoughts shift, and behaviors change, leaving you wondering how to keep your bond strong. But here's the silver lining: even as dementia takes its toll, you can still nurture and deepen your emotional connection.

Heartfelt Social Connections

- Navigate anxiety and memory loss by choosing cozy places, inviting old pals, and letting the magic of music and photos spark heartwarming conversations.

Nostalgia in Familiar Spaces

- Rediscover the power of familiar settings.

  ○ Choose places with sentimental value, creating a comforting bridge between then and now.

Old Friends, New Joy

- Invite old friends for a reunion filled with laughter and shared memories, which bring comfort.

Music and Photos as Storytellers

- Let the melody of beloved tunes and the charm of photos become storytellers. These timeless cues can stir emotions and forge connections even when words falter.

Explore Memory Care Programs for Added Support

- Explore memory care programs where supportive activities and outings create a nurturing haven for you and your loved one, fostering a bond beyond words.

Joyful Engagement for Mind, Body, and Soul

- Despite the challenges, find joy in activities that ignite the mind, nurture the body, and stir the soul.

FACILITATING ENGAGEMENT

Connecting with a loved one who has dementia can be quite a journey, filled with ups and downs. But even in the challenges lie beautiful moments of connection and reward.

Shared Music Moments

- Create a playlist of their favorite songs or tunes from their era.

  ○ Music has a unique ability to evoke memories and emotions.

- Sing along or listen together, allowing the rhythm to spark shared joy.

Memory Lane With Photo Albums

- Explore old photo albums together, reminiscing about family vacations, celebrations, and special moments.

Gentle Exercise Sessions

- Simple activities like seated stretches or a short walk can promote physical well-being and provide an opportunity for shared moments of laughter and encouragement.

Creative Arts and Crafts

- Simple projects like painting, drawing, or making personalized greeting cards can stimulate their imagination and offer a sense of accomplishment.

Cooking Together

- Cooking engages multiple senses, and familiar smells and tastes can evoke memories.

Virtual Tours and Armchair Travel

- Take virtual tours of famous landmarks or revisit places from their past.

  ○ Online platforms offer virtual experiences that can transport you both, sparking conversations and enriching your shared experiences.

Nature Connection

- Spend time outdoors, whether in a garden, a local park, or simply sitting on a porch.

  ○ Nature has a calming effect and provides a serene backdrop for conversation and shared contemplation.

Storytelling and Oral Histories

- Share stories from your life or encourage them to reminisce about their past.
- Create an oral history by recording these narratives, preserving precious memories for future reflections.

Sensory Stimulation

- Engage their senses with textured objects, scented oils, or soothing sounds.

○ These sensory experiences can be calming and offer shared relaxation and connection.

Simple Puzzle Time

- Choose puzzles with large, easy-to-handle pieces that match their cognitive abilities.

  ○ Puzzle time provides a structured yet enjoyable way to collaborate.

Always remember that patience and flexibility are key. Not every activity will hit the mark, so it's important to pay attention to their responses and make changes as needed. The aim isn't to be flawless but to foster an atmosphere where love and connection can thrive, making your time together meaningful and enriching.

EMOTIONAL CHALLENGES IN DEMENTIA CAREGIVING

As your loved one's condition progresses, you may notice their ability to express themselves and understand others slipping away. It can be tough to witness, and you might feel a whirlwind of emotions. Moments of frustration may sneak up when you find it hard to decode their needs, leaving you feeling helpless and disheartened.

Likewise, dealing with agitation or uncooperative behavior from your loved one can stir up feelings of anger or resentment. Reflecting on these moments can help you understand the complexity of your own reactions and emotions.

The communication barrier can also lead to a sense of isolation and sadness. The once cherished connection may feel distant, replaced by the struggle to understand each other.

Recognizing and grappling with these emotional hurdles is crucial to your caregiving journey. By tending to your own emotional well-being, you'll be better equipped to provide the warmth and support your loved one needs during this challenging time.

COLLABORATING WITH HEALTHCARE PROFESSIONALS

Forge a meaningful bond with your loved one's healthcare team; it's not just a step—it's a vital piece of the puzzle to ensure your loved one receives the care they deserve. Recognize your pivotal role in this journey of care. Approach interactions with empathy, understanding the hurdles they encounter.

As you stand up for your loved one, do so with resilience and compassion, ensuring their needs are addressed with respect and expertise. You're their advocate, their voice, and your presence in their care team is invaluable.

Open Communication Channels

- Establish clear and open lines of communication with healthcare professionals.
- Share information about your loved one's condition, concerns, and any changes you observe.
- Be proactive in reaching out when needed.

Active Participation in Care Planning

- Actively engage in the development of your loved one's care plan.
- Collaborate with healthcare professionals to understand treatment options, potential side effects, and any adjustments needed to enhance the quality of care.

Regularly Attend Medical Appointments

- Attend medical appointments with your loved one whenever possible.

  ○ This allows you to stay informed about their health, ask questions, and provide valuable insights that contribute to a comprehensive understanding of their well-being.

Keep an Organized Medical Record

- Maintain a comprehensive and organized medical record for your loved one.

  ○ This includes a list of medications, relevant test results, and any changes in symptoms.
  ○ Share this information with healthcare professionals for a more holistic view of their health.

Advocate for Your Loved One's Needs

- Be a strong advocate for your loved one.

  ○ Your insights are valuable in tailoring the care plan to meet their needs.

Seek Clarification on Treatment Plans

- If you have questions or uncertainties about the treatment plan, don't hesitate to seek clarification.

○ Understanding the rationale behind medical decisions can empower you to contribute more effectively to your loved one's care.

Stay Informed About Available Resources

- Stay informed about available resources and support services.
- Healthcare professionals can provide information on local agencies, support groups, and other resources to enhance the overall care experience.

Establish a Relationship of Trust

- Foster a relationship of trust with healthcare professionals.
- Share your concerns openly, listen to their expertise, and collaborate to make informed decisions about your loved one's care.

Be Proactive in Preventive Care

- Collaborate with healthcare professionals to implement preventive care measures.
- Discuss vaccination schedules, screenings, and other proactive measures contributing to your loved one's well-being.

Prioritize Your Well-Being

- Don't forget to prioritize your well-being.
- Communicate openly about any challenges you may be facing as a caregiver.

○ Healthcare professionals can offer guidance and connect you with support services to ensure you're adequately supported.

ADVOCATING FOR YOUR LOVED ONES NEEDS

As you walk the path of caregiving, advocating for your loved one's needs is more than just a task—it's a heartfelt commitment driven by love and dedication. Let compassion guide you along this journey, warming each step as you strive to provide your beloved with the best care and support.

Know Your Rights and Responsibilities

- **Rights as a Caregiver**

  ○ As the primary caregiver, you can be actively involved in your loved one's care, accessing essential information and support.

- **Responsibility to Respect**

  ○ Simultaneously, upholding your loved one's dignity, privacy, and preferences is crucial.
  ○ Familiarize yourself with relevant laws and policies that shape your role and safeguard your loved one's rights.

Communicate With Compassion

- **Clear and Respectful Language**

  ○ When discussing your loved one's needs and concerns, opt for clear, respectful, and assertive language.

○ Avoid blame or accusations, fostering an atmosphere of understanding.

- **Active Listening**

○ Actively listen to others involved in the caregiving process.
○ Acknowledge their perspectives, creating a space for collaborative and empathetic communication.

Research and Information Gathering

○ Conduct thorough research before engaging with medical professionals, family members, or service providers.
○ Gather relevant information and be well informed about your loved one's condition and needs.

- **Document Supportive Evidence**

○ Don't forget to gather important documents like medical records, care plans, or legal papers that support your case.
○ These documents clarify your loved one's situation and can help you advocate more effectively.

- **Clarify Goals and Compromises**

○ Before diving into discussions, make sure you have a clear plan.
○ Outline your goals, concerns, and areas where you're flexible.
○ Having this clarity paves the way for productive teamwork.

CLOSING THOUGHTS

In the previous chapter, we explored how important it is to foster healthy relationships as a dementia caregiver. Relationships can be a source of joy, strength, and resilience for you and your loved one. They can also help you cope with the challenges and changes that dementia brings. However, relationships are not static; they evolve and transform over time, especially as you and your loved one enter the final stage of your journey together. This stage can be emotionally intense and complex as you face the reality of losing your loved one and saying goodbye.

That's why, in the following chapter, we will explore the concept of closure and how it can help you and your loved one find peace and acceptance. I will also share tips on fostering meaningful connections and collaborations with your loved one, family, friends, and care team. These relationships can provide immense support and comfort as you and your loved one approach the end of the road together.

7

EMBRACING THE JOURNEY'S END

Grief never ends. But it changes. It is a passage, not a place to stay. Grief is not a sign of weakness nor a lack of faith; It is the price of love.

— QUEEN ELIZABETH I

As people grow older and their memory fades, it can feel like something important is slipping away. Feeling sad and missing someone can weigh on us like a heavy blanket. But it's okay to feel this way. It shows how much we care about the person we're missing. Even when things seem really tough, there are still good things to hold onto. We can remember all the good times we shared and the things that made our loved ones special. And even though they're gone, their love stays with us, shaping our lives in special ways. We can honor them by remembering the good times, the wise things they said, and the good they did in the world.

PREPARING FOR END-OF-LIFE CARE

Helping someone through dementia is like going on a tough journey. It's like sailing on rough seas, where challenges keep coming like big waves. At first, you figure out how to deal with it and find moments of happiness despite the ups and downs.

But as time goes on, things get harder and harder. Soon, you realize that the journey is almost over. This realization can be scary but also comforting at the same time, knowing that you are getting ready for the end.

As the journey continues, the person with dementia starts changing a lot physically. They might sleep more, eat differently, and move slower. Everyone handles these changes in their own way. Talking becomes more challenging for them. Frustration will grow from a lack of being able to do what they once could.

But even as things get tough, parts of who they are still shine through. Being there for emotional support becomes really important as they deal with fear, worry, and confusion.

Making decisions about their care becomes a big deal. Thinking about medical choices, planning for the future, and thinking about end-of-life care all show how much you care. Talking to doctors, lawyers, and family can help make things easier.

Websites like the Alzheimer's Society can be really helpful for people preparing for the changes. They give advice on handling the changes, dealing with legal stuff, and understanding end-of-life care.

But through all this, it's important to be kind to yourself. Accepting changes, not trying to be perfect, and just being there for your loved one show how strong you are.

Even though this time can be sad, it can also bring moments of real closeness and deep thinking. Sharing memories, singing together, and giving gentle touches create special moments to say goodbye without words—a way to honor a life well-lived. These moments, like flickering candles, keep lighting up our lives even after our loved ones are gone.

Knowing the end is near isn't giving up; it's getting ready for a peaceful end. It's about letting go of control, giving comfort and love, and cherishing the time left.

When it's time for our loved ones to go, let's remember them for the love and joy we shared, not just the tough times with dementia. By preparing for the end, we're helping them through their final days with care and understanding.

Of course, no one can say for certain how long your loved one will have to live after their diagnosis. As highlighted by Holland (2023), individuals diagnosed with dementia can live for many years, with varying life expectancies depending on the type of dementia. For instance, those with Alzheimer's disease typically live 8 to 10 years post-diagnosis. In comparison, individuals with vascular dementia may have a shorter life expectancy of around five years due to associated risks of stroke or heart attack. Patients with Lewy body dementia have an average life expectancy of 6 years post-diagnosis, with heightened risks of falls and infections, whereas frontotemporal dementia progresses more rapidly, with a life expectancy of 6 to 8 years post-diagnosis.

HOW TO CREATE A COMFORTABLE ENVIRONMENT

When your loved one is nearing the end of their life, they need to receive something called "end-of-life care." It means the help and medical care they get during this time. This care includes making them physically comfortable, caring for their feelings and emotions, meeting their spiritual needs, and helping with practical tasks.

Your role is important in ensuring your loved one feels comfortable during this tough time. Creating a comfortable environment for your dying loved one is essential for their comfort and dignity.

Here are some causes of discomfort and steps that can be taken to create a comfortable environment:

Preventing Pain

- Pain is easier to prevent than to relieve, and severe pain is hard to manage.
- Working with a doctor or nurse is important to develop a pain management plan that includes medication and non-medication strategies.

Some pain relief strategies include:

- **Palliative Medical Specialists**

  ○ These doctors know much about managing pain for sick patients.

- **Morphine**

  ○ Morphine is a strong medicine used for severe pain.
  ○ Sometimes, it's also given to help with feeling out of breath.
  ○ If your loved one is close to dying, using morphine can make them more comfortable.

Shortness of Breath

- It's common for someone at the end of their life to feel like they can't breathe well. Doctors might call this "dyspnea."
- You should raise the head of the bed, open a window, use a humidifier, or use a fan to help your loved one breathe better.
- Sometimes, medicines like morphine can also make them feel less out of breath.

Abnormal Breathing Patterns

- Sometimes, a person close to dying might have strange breathing patterns, like taking deep breaths and not breathing for a bit. It's called "Cheyne-Stokes breathing."
- They might also make noises while breathing, sometimes called a death rattle. Even though it can be alarming for family and friends, it usually doesn't bother the person who's dying.
- You can try turning them on their side or lifting their head to make them more comfortable.

Digestive Problems

- At the end of life, it's common for your loved one to have tummy issues like constipation, diarrhea, or feeling sick.
- These can happen because of illness, medicines, or other reasons.

  ○ Doctors can give medicines to help with feeling sick or unable to go to the bathroom, which can be side effects of strong pain medicines.

Skin Irritation

- Sometimes, the skin can get irritated at the end of life.

  ○ This might be due to problems such as being unable to control going to the bathroom, bedsores, or dry skin.

- If you want your loved one to avoid skin irritation, keep their skin clean and dry.

  ○ Creams and lotions that moisten the skin can also help with dry skin.

Temperature Sensitivity

- Feeling too hot or too cold can cause discomfort, dehydration, and sleep disturbances.
- Sweating and having a fever can be related, and many people with a serious illness sweat a lot and have a high temperature.
- You can do simple things to help your loved one feel better, and medicines can help once the doctor ensures there are no serious problems.

Fatigue

- Feeling tired is another common problem at the end of life. It can be caused by the illness, treatments, or emotional upset.
- Ensuring your loved one rests, eats healthy food, and drinks enough water is important to manage fatigue.

Swallowing Problems

- Sometimes, it gets hard for our loved ones to eat and drink at the end of life because of swallowing problems.
- This can lead to not having enough water and food. Illness, medicines, or other things can cause these problems.
- A speech therapist can check the swallowing problems and suggest ways to make eating and drinking easier.

When planning for the specific care needs at this stage, involving the right people is important.

Here are some suggestions on who to involve:

Healthcare Professionals

- Doctors, nurses, and social workers can provide valuable information and support during this stage.
- They can help with symptom management, pain relief, and emotional support.

Family Members and Friends

- They provide emotional support and help with meal preparation, housekeeping, and transportation.

Hospice Care Providers

- Hospice care providers can provide specialized care and support for your loved one as they approach the end of their life.
- They help you manage the symptoms, provide emotional support, and help with end-of-life planning.

When planning for the specific care needs at this stage, it is essential to consider your loved one's needs and preferences.

Symptom Management

- Your loved one may experience a range of symptoms during the later stages of the disease, including pain, agitation, and confusion.
- Working with healthcare professionals to manage these symptoms and comfort the person is important.

End-of-Life Planning

- End-of-life planning involves deciding about your loved one's care and treatment at the end of their life.
- This can include decisions about pain management, life-sustaining treatments, and hospice care.

Emotional Support

- Emotional support is important for you, your loved one, and your other family members.
- It is important to provide a supportive and caring environment that allows your loved one to express their feelings and emotions.

Creating a comfortable environment, involving the right people, and planning for the specific care needs at this stage are all important steps in caring for a dying person with dementia.

HOSPICE AND PALLIATIVE CARE

When your loved one is nearing the end of life, it's essential to understand the differences between hospice and palliative care. Hospice care aims to provide comfort and support during the final days, while palliative care focuses on improving the quality of life for individuals facing serious illnesses, regardless of life expectancy.

Palliative Care

- **When:** Available to patients at any stage of a serious illness.
- **Goals:** Aim to improve the quality of life by addressing pain, symptoms, and emotional needs.
- **Treatment:** Can be provided alongside treatments aimed at curing the illness.

Hospice Care

- **When:** Intended for the final months of life when curative treatments are no longer pursued.
- **Goals:** Focus entirely on comfort and quality of life in the end-of-life stage.
- **Treatment:** Shifts the focus from curing the illness to ensuring comfort and dignity.

Palliative Care Teams

- Work closely with patients facing serious illnesses to improve their quality of life.
- Team members, including doctors, nurses, and social workers, collaborate to provide holistic care.

- Offer comprehensive support, from pain management to emotional and spiritual guidance.
- Help with daily activities like bathing and dressing, prioritizing comfort and well-being.
- Provide counseling and bereavement services to family members and caregivers, offering a supportive shoulder to lean on.

Hospice Care Teams

- Made up of medical professionals and compassionate volunteers.
- Provide comprehensive care for those in the final stages of life, including pain management, symptom control, and emotional and spiritual support.
- Assist with daily tasks like bathing and dressing, ensuring comfort and dignity.
- Offer counseling and bereavement services to family members and caregivers, guiding them through this challenging time.

Communication With Hospice and Palliative Care Teams

- Open and honest communication is key to ensuring your loved one receives the best care possible.
- By sharing your needs and concerns, you help tailor the care to meet your loved one's wishes and preferences.
- Together, you'll prepare for end-of-life decisions, including pain and symptom management, as well as addressing emotional and spiritual needs.

COMFORT MEASURES AND PALLIATIVE CARE OPTIONS

When we're nearing the end of life with someone we care about, our primary focus is ensuring they feel comfortable and supported. As we walk alongside our loved ones during their final journey in life, ensuring their comfort and support becomes not just a priority but our utmost commitment. It's a time when every gesture and action is infused with the deep desire to ease their burdens, soothe their pains, and surround them with love and care. This dedication to their well-being encompasses not only their physical comfort but also their emotional and spiritual needs. We strive to create an environment where they feel safe, cherished, and at peace, knowing they are not alone in their journey.

Physical Comfort During the Dying Process

Pain Management

- Ensure measures are in place to address any pain your loved one may be experiencing.
- Collaborate with healthcare providers to determine the most effective pain relief methods.

Address Breathing Issues

- Work with healthcare providers to manage any breathing problems your loved one may face.
- Medication or other interventions may be used to enhance comfort.

Skin Care

- Alleviate skin irritation by implementing proper skin care measures. Use gentle and soothing methods to ensure your loved one's skin remains comfortable.

Temperature Regulation

- Attend to temperature sensitivity by ensuring the environment is conducive to your loved one's comfort.
- Adjust room temperature or provide additional blankets as needed.

Combat Fatigue

- Take steps to manage fatigue effectively.
- Allow your loved one adequate rest, and coordinate with healthcare providers to explore strategies to mitigate fatigue.

Meeting Mental and Emotional Needs During End-of-Life

Acknowledge a Range of Emotions

- Recognize that your loved one may go through various emotions like fear, anxiety, depression, and sadness.

Provide Emotional Support

- Extend emotional support to help your loved one cope with their feelings.

Explore Counseling and Therapy

- Consider counseling or therapy options to provide professional support for your loved one's mental and emotional well-being.

Be Present

- Your physical and emotional presence can offer comfort and reassurance, allowing your loved one to feel supported.

Active Listening

- Create a space where they feel heard and respected, fostering a sense of connection.

Encourage Expressing Feelings

- Encourage your loved one to express their feelings openly.

Share Positive Memories

- Discussing life, memories, and personal reflections can bring a sense of purpose and closure.

Respect Individual Coping Styles

- Respect your loved one's individual coping style and provide support tailored to their preferences.

Explore Spiritual Guidance

- Explore spiritual guidance or support if spirituality is important to your loved one.

Attending to Spiritual Needs With Respect and Compassion

Respect Beliefs and Faith

- Recognize and honor your loved one's faith or spirituality. Please show respect for their beliefs and understand that this aspect can bring comfort and solace during the end-of-life journey.

Engage in Prayer or Meditation

- Offer opportunities for prayer or meditation if your loved one finds solace in these practices.

Connect With Spiritual Leaders

- Facilitate connections with spiritual leaders or counselors who can provide guidance and support. Many find comfort in conversations with individuals who share their faith.

Provide Access to Sacred Texts

- Offer access to sacred texts or religious literature that holds significance for your loved one. Reading or listening to passages may offer comfort and a sense of connection.

Arrange for Spiritual Rituals

- If appropriate, arrange for spiritual rituals that align with your loved one's beliefs. This may include ceremonies, blessings, or other practices that bring a sense of spiritual fulfillment.

Encourage Expressing Spiritual Thoughts

- Create an open atmosphere where your loved one feels comfortable expressing their spiritual thoughts and feelings. Encourage them to share and reflect on the significance of their beliefs.

Offer Supportive Conversations

- Engage in supportive conversations about faith and spirituality. Share your thoughts if you are comfortable, fostering a connection through shared beliefs.

Respect Individual Spiritual Journey

- Respect that each individual's spiritual journey is unique. Be mindful of your loved one's beliefs and preferences, ensuring their spiritual needs are met with understanding and compassion.

Supporting Practical Needs With Compassion and Dignity

Assist With Daily Tasks

- Offer assistance with essential daily tasks such as bathing, dressing, and eating. Recognize the importance of these activities in maintaining your loved one's comfort and well-being.

Provide Gentle and Compassionate Care

- Approach practical tasks with compassion and gentleness. Your caregiving should prioritize your loved one's comfort, fostering an environment of trust and respect.

Respect Personal Dignity

- Ensure that your loved one's dignity is maintained throughout every task. Respect their autonomy and preferences, allowing them to retain a sense of control over their personal care.

Maintain Open Communication

- Keep communication open regarding practical tasks. Discuss preferences and any specific needs your loved one may have, ensuring their comfort and dignity are prioritized.

Create a Comfortable Environment

- Establish a comfortable and private environment for practical tasks. This can enhance your loved one's sense of security and provide a positive caregiving experience.

Coordinate With Healthcare Professionals

- Collaborate with healthcare professionals to ensure practical tasks align with your loved one's medical and care plan.

Offer Emotional Support

- Recognize that practical tasks may be emotionally challenging for your loved one. Offer emotional support and reassurance, acknowledging the importance of their well-being beyond the physical aspect.

Celebrate Achievements

- Acknowledge and celebrate achievements in daily tasks. No matter how small, every accomplishment contributes to your loved one's overall well-being and achievement.

When considering palliative care for your loved one, it's vital to have heartfelt conversations with the care team. They're here to support you, so don't hesitate to share your worries and needs. Palliative care is all about improving the quality of life by easing symptoms. And guess what? Other supportive options like respite care and hospice care might also be helpful. It's about finding what suits your loved one best; your voice in this decision is incredibly important.

If you need a place to start, here are some of the questions you may want to ask your care provider:

- What services are included in palliative care?
- How can palliative care help me or my loved one?

- Who provides palliative care, and where is it available?
- How do I access palliative care services?
- Will my insurance cover palliative care?
- How can I communicate my wishes and preferences to my care team?
- How can I manage pain and other symptoms?
- How can I address emotional and spiritual needs?
- How can I prepare for my loved one's passing?

EMOTIONAL SUPPORT AND CLOSURE

There's no denying you're in for a tough, emotional ride. While caring for someone during a difficult illness, there is no denying you will feel so many different emotions all at once.

You might be sad about the person they used to be. It is human nature to feel bad, thinking you're not doing enough for your loved one or could do better. There will be days when you will be exhausted from caring for them, but that shouldn't surprise you. Caregiving is a lot of work, both physically and emotionally. You might become upset or angry with grief as you get ready for the sad loss that's around the corner.

All these ups and downs can isolate you. There will also be days when you will feel helpless. But it's important to know that feeling this way is okay. Don't forget to ask for help when you need it. You're not alone in this.

The Importance of Emotional Support

Supporting someone through dementia is really important for both the person with dementia and the caregiver. It can be tough sometimes to see changes in your loved one and deal with the challenges of taking care of them every day. But it's totally okay to feel overwhelmed and to ask for help from friends, family, or other caregivers. Talking about how you feel can make things easier and help you connect with others who are going through similar experiences.

As a caregiver, you play a significant role in making the person with dementia feel comfortable and safe. Creating a calm and familiar environment is important, especially as the disease worsens. Doing simple things like holding their hand, saying kind words, or playing their favorite music can bring them comfort when things feel uncertain. Good communication is also key for providing emotional support. Sometimes, you might need to use non-verbal cues or show empathy when words are hard to understand. Staying in the present moment, finding new ways to connect, and cherishing the time you spend together all help keep your emotions in check.

On this journey, you'll find strength in supporting each other emotionally. Seeing the person behind the disease and recognizing their resilience and dignity brings you closer together. It's all about creating a caring and understanding atmosphere and navigating through tough emotions together. Remember, you're not just a caregiver—you're also a source of comfort, making a loving space that lifts both your spirits and theirs.

Caring for Your Emotional Well-Being

Remember, taking care of your emotional well-being is necessary, especially during this preparation for the end of life. It allows you to provide the best care for your loved one.

Acknowledge Your Feelings

- Recognize and accept the emotions you're going through, like grief and anxiety.

Connect With Support

- Reach out to people who get what you're dealing with.

Take Regular Breaks

- Schedule downtime to recharge.

Set Realistic Expectations

- Be realistic about what you can handle.

Prioritize Self-Care

- Take care of yourself. Get enough rest, eat well, and do things that bring you comfort.

Consider Professional Help

- If you need it, talk to a professional. It can be hugely helpful to have someone with whom you can discuss your feelings and coping strategies.

Stay Informed

- Learn about what to expect in the end-of-life process. Knowing more can give you a sense of control and reduce uncertainty.

Celebrate Meaningful Moments

- Cherish special moments with your loved one.

Maintain Connection

- Stay connected with your loved one. Be present and share comforting moments, even in tough times.

Delegate Responsibilities

- Don't be afraid to ask for help. Get support from friends, family, or professionals. Sharing the load is crucial during this emotionally challenging period.

NAVIGATING THREE TYPES OF GOODBYES

Saying goodbye to someone you love can be one of the toughest parts of being a caregiver. Dr. David Solie, a specialist in understanding aging, talks about three kinds of goodbyes that can help you navigate this difficult time (*The Three Goodbyes,* 2014).

Goodbye of Separation

- In earlier stages, when your loved one still recognizes you, say goodbye as if you'll meet again soon.
- Maintain a connection and offer reassurance.

Goodbye of Release

- As dementia progresses to later stages, recognition may fade. Acknowledge that your loved one is moving to a different place.

- It's a way for you to let go and recognize the inevitable journey.

Goodbye of Ritual

- Applicable at any stage, create a meaningful farewell with prayers, songs, readings, or significant activities for you and your loved one.

Coming to terms with the reality that your loved one is nearing the end of their life is a big step to take. It's important to gather information, talk openly with others, reach out to your support system, and make time to cope better and be ready to provide care.

COPING WITH GRIEF, LOSS, AND BEREAVEMENT

Feeling sad when you lose someone is normal, especially for caregivers dealing with people with dementia because it lasts a long time. To help yourself through it, try talking about and showing your feelings, remembering the person with special ceremonies or pictures, finding meaning in what you did for them, doing things that make you happy, and looking for hope and good things.

Reminiscing: A Path to Connection

Experiencing the slow fading of memories, personality, and identity in dementia can be tough for caregivers like you. Reminiscing, which means talking about and sharing past experiences, is a helpful way to honor and stay connected with the person with dementia. It helps their brain work better, makes them happier, strengthens their connection, and gives them a sense of who they are.

When you're reminiscing, be flexible, patient, and respectful. Use little clues to help them remember things, ask questions that don't have yes or no answers, understand and accept their feelings, let them take the lead in the conversation, and most importantly, focus on enjoying the moment together instead of checking their memory. Doing these things creates an environment that brings you closer to the person you love and care about.

Honoring Their Memory: A Guide to Posthumous Tribute

The path of dementia often ends with the loss of someone you love, and dealing with the sadness can be hard. Honoring the memory of the person who passed away is a way to keep their spirit alive and find comfort in the middle of your grief. You can do different things, like making memory boxes, planting trees, giving to charity, joining memory walks, sharing stories, lighting candles, creating memorials, making scrapbooks, or writing letters. These options give caregivers like you various ways to show love and remember the life of the person you cared for (Thurston, 2011).

Grief Counseling: A Compass in the Mourning Process

If you're feeling weighed down by grief, don't hesitate to seek out counseling—it can truly make a huge difference. Grief counseling is like having a caring guide by your side as you navigate the stormy seas of losing someone close to you. It's a safe and understanding place to express your feelings and work through your emotional challenges.

SAMHSA and Online Resources

- SAMHSA and other reputable organizations offer valuable support.
- Explore their online and offline resources to find guidance tailored to your needs.

National Mental Health Groups Like NAMI

- Connect with national mental health groups, such as NAMI, where understanding ears and compassionate hearts are ready to listen and assist on your journey.

Specialized Grief Support Services (HealGrief)

- Services like HealGrief specialize in offering dedicated grief support.
- Their tailored approach can provide solace and understanding during this challenging time.

Licensed Counselors Through the American Counseling Association (ACA)

- Engage with licensed counselors affiliated with organizations like ACA.
- Their expertise can offer personalized guidance and support as you navigate through your grief.

These options aren't just paths to lean on for emotional support; they're shining lights of hope to kickstart the process of healing. Remember, reaching out for help is a brave step toward acknowledging your pain and making room for healing.

Being there for someone on the dementia journey is emotionally demanding. People play a huge role in shaping this story, from facing the challenges of the disease's progression to saying goodbye and coping with what follows. Offering and receiving emotional support, acknowledging and embracing grief, and finding meaningful ways to honor and stay connected with the person with dementia—both during and after their journey—are incredibly important aspects of this voyage.

MIXED FEELINGS OF CAREGIVERS

As your caregiving role shifts, whether due to the passing of the person you've been caring for, you might find yourself grappling with a mix of emotions. The conclusion of this journey can stir up a range of feelings like relief, grief, guilt, and uncertainty. You might even feel torn about feeling relieved now that your responsibilities have come to an end.

The grieving process might extend beyond mourning the loss of your loved one to include feelings of losing your sense of identity, purpose, and the familiar routines associated with your caregiving role. It's important to recognize and accept these complex emotions as a crucial first step (Dardis, 2016). Remember, these feelings are natural and don't diminish the love and dedication you've shown.

It's equally vital to find healthy ways to express these emotions. Whether it's having heartfelt conversations with trusted friends, pouring your thoughts into a journal, or seeking support from a professional counselor, giving voice to your feelings can help release emotional tension and guide you toward healing and moving forward.

Rediscovering Identity

Now, it's time for you to rediscover your identity outside the caregiving role. You might have put aside your needs, interests, and goals while dedicating yourself to your loved one. This is your chance to explore both old and new interests, reconnect with relationships that may have been strained, and re-establish your values, beliefs, and strengths. Take this opportunity to focus on yourself and what brings you fulfillment and joy.

Strategies for Rediscovery

- Engage in enjoyable activities.
- Learn new skills or knowledge.
- Reconnect with family and friends.
- Seek personal or professional development.
- Practice self-care and self-compassion.
- Reflect on the caregiving experience and its impact.

Applying Skills and Strengths

Now, it's time to put into action all the valuable skills and strengths you've gained from your experiences. You might need to fully grasp the extent of the knowledge and achievements you've amassed. Pause for a moment to acknowledge the treasure trove of skills you've built and think about how they can make a positive difference, not just in your own life but also in your communities. Your unique journey has armed you with powerful tools; it's time to use them to shape your future endeavors.

Ways to Apply Skills and Strengths

- Identify transferable skills gained through caregiving.
- Share caregiving experiences through writing, speaking, or mentoring.
- Advocate for caregivers' needs and rights.
- Pursue a career or education in a related field.
- Volunteer or work for caregiving-related organizations.
- Use caregiving experiences as a source of inspiration and resilience.

I wish to guide you through the intricate process of transitioning from the caregiving role to a new phase of life. By acknowledging mixed feelings, rediscovering identity, and applying skills and strengths, you are ready for healing, self-discovery, and personal growth.

STORIES OF STRENGTH

Meet Tracey Clayton, a remarkable caregiver who dedicated nine years of her life to caring for her aunt. Tracey's journey taught her that caregiving requires an abundance of time, dedication, and patience. It's a roller-coaster ride filled with both rewarding moments and tough challenges as the person's abilities decline. But amidst the struggles, Tracey discovered effective ways to support someone with dementia, even when they resist help. Simple words, establishing routines, and avoiding arguments became her allies in navigating the journey.

Early detection and treatment of memory issues can significantly enhance the quality of life for those affected. Alzheimer's disease, the leading cause of dementia, accounts for a substantial portion of cases. As a caregiver, it's crucial to prioritize self-care and seek support from loved ones, friends, or support groups. Remember, you're not alone in this journey, and taking care of yourself is just as vital as caring for your loved one.

Then there's Kathy Siggins, whose husband Gene battled Alzheimer's disease for 12 long years. Kathy's caregiving experience was all-consuming, but she found solace and strength in support groups. These gatherings provided a lifeline for Kathy, connecting her with others who understood the unique challenges of caregiving. With the guidance of experts like Dr. Constantine Lyketsos, Kathy navigated the complex terrain of caregiving, finding invaluable resources and support along the way.

Following Gene's passing, Kathy transformed her grief into action, becoming a passionate advocate for Alzheimer's research. Together with fellow advocates, she spearheaded the creation of a fundraising stamp that generated over $70 million for research. Kathy's journey exemplifies the resilience and compassion of caregivers who impact the lives of their loved ones and the broader community.

Lastly, there's Kim, whose love story with Jeffrey took an unexpected turn when he began showing signs of cognitive decline. Despite the challenges, Kim became Jeffrey's primary caregiver while juggling two jobs and caring for her parents. She grappled with a whirlwind of emotions, from stress and guilt to the fear of losing her beloved husband. Seeking support from a counselor, prioritizing self-care, and cherishing moments with Jeffrey helped Kim navigate the turbulent waters of caregiving. Her story epitomizes unconditional love and courage in the face of adversity, offering hope and inspiration to fellow caregivers on similar journeys.

CLOSING THOUGHTS

As you close the chapter on your caregiving journey, remember that it's not just an ending but the start of something new. You've poured love, strength, and wisdom into caring for your loved one, making their last days filled with peace and purpose. Now, it's time to honor their life and the legacy they've left behind while stepping into your future with hope and gratitude.

THE TORCHBEARER'S PARTING GIFT

Now that you've armed yourself with the knowledge and strategies to navigate the world of dementia caregiving, it's your turn to light the way for others. By sharing your genuine thoughts about this book on Amazon, you guide fellow caregivers to the support and wisdom they seek, perpetuating the cycle of learning and compassion.

Leaving your review is more than just feedback; it's a beacon for other caregivers seeking guidance and understanding. Your insights can help them find the same solace and practical advice you discovered, continuing the legacy of care and support that defines our community.

Thank you for your invaluable contribution. The journey of dementia caregiving is enriched and preserved through the sharing of our collective knowledge—and by participating, you play a pivotal role in that mission.

SCAN ME

CONCLUSION

As you undertake this challenging yet meaningful responsibility of caring for someone with dementia, let this toolkit be your glowing torch, helping make your path safer and clearer with its practical solutions and emotional support.

Inside this toolkit, you have discovered a treasure trove of insights. From understanding the stages of dementia to developing coping strategies for the emotional toll it can take, each chapter equips you with the tools to navigate the challenges confidently. No matter how high the highs or how low the lows, you have a trusty guide to lean on through it all.

But this book isn't just about information put 'on' a page. It was a wake-up call to remember to take care of yourself, too. Remember, caregiving can be demanding, so it's crucial to prioritize your well-being.

Now, you will always have these practical tips and exercises at your fingertips if you need help recharging your battery. Remember, when you learn to properly care for your mental health and maintain your energy levels, you can continue providing the best care for your loved one.

Moreover, the toolkit explores the importance of communication and connection in caregiving relationships. From fostering meaningful connections with your loved one to maintaining open lines of communication with medical professionals, it offers guidance on nurturing relationships and promoting a sense of belonging.

As you journeyed through the toolkit, you have picked up numerous resources and tools to enhance your effectiveness as a caregiver. Each tool empowers you in your caregiving role, from checklists and templates to practical exercises and reflection prompts.

By understanding and managing your loved one's behavioral changes, you are equipped with strategies to recognize and respond to the challenging behaviors associated with dementia.

This toolkit also addressed practical aspects like budgeting, planning for the future, and navigating legal and financial matters. This provided you with valuable insights into managing the various aspects of caregiving.

Finally, the toolkit offered preparation and guidance for the end-of-life stages. It provided insight into coping with the challenges associated with this phase, helping you find meaning and closure at the end of your loved one's life.

The ultimate goal is not only to handle the complexities of dementia caregiving but to emerge from the experience as a stronger, more empowered version of yourself. This means facing the role with compassion, courage, and resilience, fostering a positive and fulfilling caregiving experience.

Meet Sarah, a devoted daughter caring for her mother, who was recently diagnosed with dementia. At first, Sarah felt overwhelmed by the new responsibilities and challenges of caregiving. She struggled to understand her mother's changing behaviors and felt emotionally drained from the constant worry and stress.

Feeling lost and unsure where to turn, Sarah stumbled upon *The Dementia Caregiver's Toolkit*. As she flipped through the pages, she felt a sense of relief wash over her. The practical advice and heartfelt stories shared within the book resonated deeply with her, providing her with the guidance and support she desperately needed.

Armed with the tools and strategies outlined in the toolkit, Sarah felt more confident in her caregiving role. She learned how to create a structured routine for her mother, manage challenging behaviors with patience and understanding, and prioritize her self-care to prevent burnout.

With each passing day, Sarah noticed positive changes in herself and her mother. Their relationship grew stronger as they found new ways to connect and communicate. Sarah felt empowered knowing that she had the resources she needed to navigate the ups and downs of dementia caregiving.

Inspired by her own experience, Sarah decided to share *The Dementia Caregiver's Toolkit* with her best friend, Emily, who was also caring for her aging father with dementia. Seeing how much the toolkit had helped her, Sarah knew that Emily would also benefit from its guidance and support.

Encouraged by Sarah's recommendation, Emily eagerly dove into the toolkit and soon found herself feeling more equipped to handle the challenges of caregiving. Like Sarah, she discovered valuable insights and practical tools that helped her navigate the complexities of dementia care with confidence and compassion.

Sarah and Emily formed a support network, sharing their experiences, offering encouragement, and lending a listening ear whenever needed. They realized that by sharing *The Dementia Caregiver's Toolkit*, they had helped themselves and positively impacted someone else's caregiving journey.

So, if, like Sarah, you've found value in *The Dementia Caregiver's Toolkit*, consider paying it forward by sharing it with someone else who may benefit from its guidance and support. By doing so, you'll not only be helping them navigate their caregiving journey but also spreading kindness and support within your caregiving community.

Remember, we're all in this together, and by supporting each other, we can make the caregiving journey a little bit easier and more rewarding for everyone.

REFERENCES

A caregiver's checklist for your loved one suffering from dementia. (2019, July 25). Oxford Home Health Care. https://www.oxford-healthcare.com/blog/2019/7/25/a-caregivers-checklist-for-daily-care-of-your-loved-one-suffering-from-dementia

Accepting the diagnosis. (2021). Alzheimer's Disease and Dementia. https://www.alz.org/help-support/caregiving/stages-behaviors/accepting_the_diagnosis

Alexy, J. (2018, August 7). *Setting boundaries as a caregiver | Resource | Aegis Living.* Áegis Living Assisted Living Memory Care. https://www.aegisliving.com/resource-center/set-boundaries-as-a-caregiver/

Allen, J., Caiquo, J., Sumner, M., Tawil, A., & Mele, J. (2021). *Environmental Modifications for Dementia Care.* Stanbridge Repository. https://repository.stanbridge.edu/95/1/MSOT010.10.pdf

Allen, K. (2015, May 25). *Activities to get the Alzheimer's and dementia patient engaged.* BrightFocus Foundation. https://www.brightfocus.org/alzheimers/article/activities-get-alzheimers-and-dementia-patient-engaged

Allen, K. (2016, April 20). *Three experienced Alzheimer's and Dementia caregivers share their stories and lessons.* BrightFocus Foundation. https://www.brightfocus.org/alzheimers/article/three-experienced-alzheimers-and-dementia-caregivers-share-their-stories-and

Alzheimer's caregiving: Changes in communication skills. (2017a). National Institute on Aging. https://www.nia.nih.gov/health/alzheimers-caregiving-changes-communication-skills

Azevedo, M. C. D. de, Charchat-Fichman, H., & Damazio, V. M. M. (2021). Environmental interventions to support orientation and social engagement of people with Alzheimer's disease. *Dementia & Neuropsychologia, 15*(4), 510–523. https://doi.org/10.1590/1980-57642021dn15-040012

Bathing, dressing, and grooming: Alzheimer's caregiving tips. (2017b). National Institute on Aging. https://www.nia.nih.gov/health/bathing-dressing-and-grooming-alzheimers-caregiving-tips

Betcher, B. (2018, March 2). *9 ways to honor a loved one who has passed.* CaringBridge. https://www.caringbridge.org/resources/9-ways-remember-loved-one-passed/

Botek, A.-M. (2013, March 26). *Why a daily routine is helpful for people with dementia.*

Aging Care. https://www.agingcare.com/articles/daily-routine-for-people-with-dementia-156855.htm

Braun, A. (2021, June 14). *The 10 best online grief support groups of 2021*. Healthline. https://www.healthline.com/health/mental-health/online-grief-support-groups

Brauner, R. (2020, March 5). *Caregiving & conflict with family members*. OneOp. https://oneop.org/2020/03/05/caregiving-conflict-with-family-members/

Build an emergency fund. (2022, June 29). Investopedia. https://www.investopedia.com/personal-finance/how-to-build-emergency-fund/

Caregivers: Be realistic, think positive. (2021, October 28). American Heart Association. https://www.heart.org/en/health-topics/caregiver-support/caregivers-be-realistic-think-positive

Caregivers share: Tips for bathing, grooming, and dressing. (2023, April 11). Alzheimer's Caregivers Network. https://alzheimerscaregivers.org/2023/04/11/caregivers-share-tips-for-bathing-grooming-and-dressing/

Caregiver statistics: Demographics. (2016). Family Caregiver Alliance. https://www.caregiver.org/resource/caregiver-statistics-demographics/

Caregiver statistics: Work and caregiving. (2016, May 10). Family Caregiver Alliance. https://www.caregiver.org/resource/caregiver-statistics-work-and-caregiving/

Cecchini, C. (2023, June). *7 signs that death may be near in someone with dementia*. GoodRx. https://www.goodrx.com/conditions/dementia/signs-death-is-near-dementia

Changes in behavior. (2021, August 12). Alzheimer's Society. https://www.alzheimers.org.uk/about-dementia/symptoms-and-diagnosis/symptoms/behaviour-changes

Christiansen, S. (2019, January 19). *How to create a checklist and daily care plan for dementia*. Alzheimers. https://www.alzheimers.net/checklist-and-daily-care-plan-for-dementia

Cook, C. (2021, March 16). *Six ways to build a positive mindset as a carer*. Mobilise. https://www.mobiliseonline.co.uk/post/6-ways-to-build-a-positive-mindset-as-a-carer

Cramer, L. (n.d.). *Dealing with resistance to care*. Alzheimer's Association. https://www.alz.org/media/cacentral/dementia-care-41-dealing-with-resistance-to-care.pdf

Creating a calming, helpful home for people with dementia. (2022, October 6). Healthdirect Australia. https://www.healthdirect.gov.au/creating-a-calming-home-for-people-with-dementia

Daily care plan. (2020a). Alzheimer's Disease and Dementia. https://www.alz.org/help-support/caregiving/daily-care/daily-care-plan

Damico, A. (2015, October 19). *Medicaid's role for people with dementia*. KFF. https://

www.kff.org/mental-health/issue-brief/medicaids-role-for-people-with-dementia/

Dardis, S. (2016, March 8). *Adjusting to life after caring for a loved one with a serious illness.* Hospice of the Red River Valley. https://www.hrrv.org/blog/adjusting-to-life-after-caring-for-a-loved-one-with-a-serious-illness/

Davis, J. (2022, February 22). *Understanding the costs of dementia care.* North River Home Care. https://www.northriverhc.com/understanding-the-costs-of-dementia-care/

Dementia. (2023, March 15). World Health Organization. https://www.who.int/news-room/fact-sheets/detail/dementia

Dementia daily care plan & checklist. (n.d.). Visiting Angels. https://www.visitingangels.com/omaha/articles/dementia-daily-care-plan-checklist/15757

Dementia - Behavior changes. (n.d.). Better Health Victoria. https://www.betterhealth.vic.gov.au/health/conditionsandtreatments/dementia-behaviour-changes#

Dementia - Communication. (2012). Better Health Channel. https://www.betterhealth.vic.gov.au/health/ConditionsAndTreatments/dementia-communication

Dressing and grooming. (2019). Alzheimer's Disease and Dementia. https://www.alz.org/help-support/caregiving/daily-care/dressing-grooming

Desai, A. K., & Grossberg, G. T. (2001). Recognition and management of behavioral disturbances in dementia. *Primary Care Companion to the Journal of Clinical Psychiatry, 3*(3), 93–109. https://doi.org/10.4088/pcc.v03n0301

Donohue, M. (2022, September 1). *The value of social support for caregivers.* Blue Moon Senior Counseling. https://bluemoonseniorcounseling.com/the-value-of-social-support-for-caregivers/

Dreher, B. S. (2017). Creating a comfort environment at end-of-life in critical care: A review. *Journal of Intensive and Critical Care, 03*(02). https://doi.org/10.21767/2471-8505.100081

Estrada, R. (2022). Listen and you will see the person through the dementia. *Journal for Person-Oriented Research, 7*(2), 88–97. https://doi.org/10.17505/jpor.2021.23891

Farrell, E. (2016, November 9). *Start the long term care conversation.* LTC Consumer. https://ltcconsumer.com/start-long-term-care-conversation/

5 practical ways caregivers can advocate for their loved one. (2022, February 12). Violet https://blog.violet.org.au/en/resources/practical-ways-to-advocate

5 steps to build an emergency fund. (2022, February 4). Securian Financial. https://www.securian.com/insights-tools/articles/5-steps-to-building-an-emergency-fund.html

Ford-Martin, P. (2022, August 22). *Types of dementia.* WebMD. https://www.webmd.com/alzheimers/alzheimers-dementia

4 reasons why long-term care planning is important. (2023, October 22). Elder Care Alliance. https://eldercarealliance.org/blog/long-term-care-planning-importance/

Fowler, K. (2019, August 26). *The importance of self-care for caregivers.* A Place for Mom. https://www.aplaceformom.com/caregiver-resources/articles/the-importance-of-self-care-for-caregivers

Freeman, A. (2023, June 9). *12 tips for balancing your life as a family caregiver.* LoveToKnow. https://www.lovetoknow.com/life/aging/balance-life-as-family-caregiver

Gillespie, C., & 2021. (2023, November 9). *Grief support groups can help you process a loss—Here's how to find one near you.* Health. https://www.health.com/mind-body/grief-support-groups

Gipple, C. (2023, May 1). *Which long term care option is the best? | Broker World.* Broker World Mag. https://brokerworldmag.com/which-long-term-care-option-is-the-best/

Gottschalk, S., Neubert, L., König, H.-H., & Brettschneider, C. (2021). Balancing care demands and personal needs: A typology on the reconciliation of informal dementia care with personal life based on narrative interviews. *Dementia,* 147130122110083. https://doi.org/10.1177/14713012211008306

Green, M. (2019). *You can't go home again: The story of a daughter and caregiver.* Alzheimer's Disease and Dementia. https://www.alz.org/blog/alz/december-2019/you-can-t-go-home-again-the-story-of-a-daughter-a

H, J. (2021, September 1). *Caregiver mental health: The importance of you.* Cerebral Palsy Research Network. https://cprn.org/caregiver-mental-health-the-importance-of-you/

Hallstrom, L. (2022, October 18). *The 7 stages of dementia & symptoms.* A Place for Mom. https://www.aplaceformom.com/caregiver-resources/articles/dementia-stages

Hansard, S. (2021, February 17). *7 lessons learned about caring for someone with dementia | Alzheimer's Society.* Alzheimer's Society. https://www.alzheimers.org.uk/blog/7-lessons-learned-caring-for-someone-dementia

Heerema, E. (2023, November 28). *9 care options for people living with dementia.* Verywell Health. https://www.verywellhealth.com/resource-guide-9-care-options-for-people-living-with-dementia-4084379

Herke, M., Fink, A., Langer, G., Wustmann, T., Watzke, S., Hanff, A.-M., & Burckhardt, M. (2018). Environmental and behavioural modifications for improving food and fluid intake in people with dementia. *Cochrane Database of Systematic Reviews, 7*(7). https://doi.org/10.1002/14651858.cd011542.pub2

Hinckley, M. P. (1999). *Glimpses Into the Life and Heart of Marjorie Pay Hinckley.* Deseret Book Co.

Holland, K. (2023, June 28). *Understanding the end-of-life signs for dementia care.* Healthline. https://www.healthline.com/health/dementia/dementia-stages-end-of-life

How to cope with the impact of caregiving on relationships with others. (2022, January 5). Careforth. https://careforth.com/blog/caregiving-can-impact-your-relationships-with-family-and-friends-heres-how-to-cope/

How to create a peaceful at-home hospice for your loved one. (2017, May 1). Home Advisor. https://www.homeadvisor.com/r/create-peaceful-at-home-hospice/

How to support a person with dementia to get dressed or change clothes. (2021). Alzheimer's Society. https://www.alzheimers.org.uk/get-support/daily-living/getting-dressed-changing-clothes

Huang, J. (2023, February). *Behavioral and psychologic symptoms of dementia - Neurologic disorders.* MSD Manual Professional Edition. https://www.msdmanuals.com/professional/neurologic-disorders/delirium-and-dementia/behavioral-and-psychologic-symptoms-of-dementia

Hudson, L. (2017, February 2). *Maintaining comfort in end of life care.* Innova Care Concepts. https://www.innovacareconcepts.com/en/blog/maintaining-comfort-in-end-of-life-care/

Involving people living with dementia in decisions about care. (2018). National Institute for Health and Care Excellence (NICE). https://www.ncbi.nlm.nih.gov/books/NBK536494/

Jones, K. (2017, July 25). *What are your strengths as a caregiver?* Hospital News. https://hospitalnews.com/what-are-your-strengths-as-a-caregiver/

Joshi, P., Tampi, R., & Srinivasan, S. (2020). Managing behavioral and psychological symptoms of dementia in the era of boxed warnings. *The American Journal of Geriatric Psychiatry, 28*(4), S29. https://doi.org/10.1016/j.jagp.2020.01.055

Kennedy, S. (2023, April 26). *Dementia care: 6 tips to overcome challenging family dynamics - Positive Approach to Care.* Positive Approach to Care. https://teepasnow.com/blog/dementia-care-6-tips-to-overcome-challenging-family-dynamics/

Keys to a successful family caregiver meeting. (2020, February 11). Independence4Senior. https://www.independence4seniors.com/blog/keys-to-a-successful-family-caregiver-meeting/

Kim's story: An Alzheimer's caregiver. (2023, March 1). Roche Diagnostics. https://diagnostics.roche.com/us/en/article-listing/kim-borghoff-alzheimer-caregiver.html

Lankford, K. (2023, August). *Does Medicare cover dementia and Alzheimer's drugs?* AARP. https://www.aarp.org/health/medicare-qa-tool/does-medicare-cover-dementia.html

Liles, M. (2021, January 29). *These 50 inspirational quotes for family caregivers will get you through tough days.* Parade. https://parade.com/1004993/marynliles/care giver-quotes/

Lindauer, A., Sexson, K., & Harvath, T. A. (2017). Medication management for people with dementia. *American Journal of Nursing, 117*(2), 60–64. https://doi. org/10.1097/01.NAJ.0000512300.41511.9d

Logan, B. (2016). *Caregiver's guide to understanding dementia behaviors.* Family Caregiver Alliance. https://www.caregiver.org/resource/caregivers-guide-understanding-dementia-behaviors/

Managing behavioral and psychological symptoms of dementia. (2015). Department of Health Victoria. https://www.health.vic.gov.au/patient-care/managing-behav ioural-and-psychological-symptoms-of-dementia

Managing legal affairs for someone with dementia. (2023, August 18). NHS. https:// www.nhs.uk/conditions/dementia/care-and-support/legal-issues/

Managing medicines for a person with Alzheimer's. (2017). National Institute on Aging. https://www.nia.nih.gov/health/managing-medicines-person-alzheimers

Managing the behavioral and psychological symptoms of dementia. (2020). BPAC NZ. https://bpac.org.nz/2020/bpsd.aspx

Malzone, L. (2022a, March 8). *Does Medicare provide coverage for dementia.* Medigap. https://www.medigap.com/faqs/medicare-coverage-dementia/

Malzone, L. (2022b, August 18). *Medicare coverage for beneficiaries with Alzheimer's disease.* Medigap. https://www.medigap.com/faqs/medicare-coverage-for-alzheimers/

Medicare. (2020). Alzheimer's Disease and Dementia. https://www.alz.org/help-support/caregiving/financial-legal-planning/medicare

Medication safety. (2019). Alzheimer's Disease and Dementia. https://www.alz.org/ help-support/caregiving/safety/medication-safety

Morrey, M. (2021, December 9). *How to reclaim your identity after being a cancer care-giver.* Children's Cancer Research Fund. https://childrenscancer.org/how-to-reclaim-your-identity-after-being-a-cancer-caregiver/

Morrisette, S. (2021, July 30). *12 top tips: Effective time management for caregivers.* Smartcare Software. https://smartcaresoftware.com/news/12-top-tips-effec tive-time-management-for-caregivers/

Nall, R. (2017, January 5). *10 types of dementia.* Healthline Media. https://www. healthline.com/health/types-dementia

Nazarko, L. (2006). Creating the ideal home for people with dementia. *Nursing and Residential Care, 8*(5), 221–223. https://doi.org/10.12968/nrec.2006.8.5.20932

Neville, J. (2013, July 17). *Holding a family meeting.* Family Caregiver Alliance. https://www.caregiver.org/resource/holding-family-meeting/

Nichols, A. (2021, March 16). *23 best caregiver support groups online and in-person.* A

Place for Mom. https://www.aplaceformom.com/caregiver-resources/articles/caregiver-support-groups

Non-verbal communication and dementia. (2022a, January 19). Alzheimer's Society. https://www.alzheimers.org.uk/about-dementia/symptoms-and-diagnosis/symptoms/non-verbal-communication-and-dementia

Nurse, N. (2021, December 13). *Finding balance in life as an Alzheimer's caregiver.* Alzheimer's Disease. https://alzheimersdisease.net/living/find-balance-in-life

Oh, S., Yu, M., Ryu, Y. M., Kim, H., & Lee, H. (2019). Changes in family dynamics in caregiving for people with dementia in South Korea: A qualitative meta-synthesis study. *Qualitative Health Research, 30*(1), 60–72. https://doi.org/10.1177/1049732319871254

On the front lines: Primary care physicians and Alzheimer's care in America. (2023). Alzheimer's Association. https://www.alz.org/media/Documents/alzheimers-facts-and-figures.pdf

100 caregiver quotes. (2020, June 1). Know Your Archetypes. https://knowyourarchetypes.com/caregiver-quotes/

Orestis, C. (2022, April 1). *Long-term care planning: Caring for loved ones.* Retirement Genius. https://retirementgenius.com/2022/04/01/discussing-long-term-care-options-with-your-loved-ones/

Pahl, L. (2023, July 9). *How to help someone with dementia cope with a death.* Caregiver. https://caregiver.com/articles/dementia-cope-death/

Palliative care: What it is & what's included. (2022, April 22). Cleveland we Clinic. https://my.clevelandclinic.org/health/articles/22850-palliative-care

Parker, T. (2021, November 16). *Here's how to choose a long-term care facility for your loved ones.* The Balance. https://www.thebalancemoney.com/how-to-choose-a-long-term-care-facility-4174494

Pedersen, T. (2023, April 10). *Average monthly cost of memory care and ways to save.* Healthline. https://www.healthline.com/health/what-is-the-average-monthly-cost-for-memory-care

Perry, E. (2022, September 7). *6 self-care tips for caregivers.* Betterup. https://www.betterup.com/blog/self-care-for-caregivers

Personal stories of caregivers, families and professionals. (2020). Alzheimer's Disease and Dementia. https://www.alz.org/wi/helping-you/personal-stories

Planning for care costs. (2020). Alzheimer's Disease and Dementia. https://www.alz.org/help-support/caregiving/financial-legal-planning/planning-for-care-costs

Protecting your personal relationship as a family caregiver. (2020, July 15). CaraVita. https://www.caravitahomecare.com/protecting-your-personal-relationship-as-a-family-caregiver/

Providing care and comfort at the end of life. (2022, November 17). National Institute on Aging. https://www.nia.nih.gov/health/end-life/providing-care-and-comfort-end-life

Recognizing when someone is reaching the end of their life. (2019). Alzheimer's Society. https://www.alzheimers.org.uk/get-support/help-dementia-care/recognising-when-someone-reaching-end-their-life

Reed-Guy, L. (2013, August 27). *The stages of dementia.* Healthline Media. https://www.healthline.com/health/dementia/stages

Reminiscence for people with dementia. (2020, October) Social Care Institute for Excellence. https://www.scie.org.uk/dementia/living-with-dementia/keeping-active/reminiscence.asp

Rifkin, R. (2019, May 22). *7 ways to honor a loved one's memory.* Next Avenue. https://www.nextavenue.org/honor-loved-ones-memory/

Robinson, L., & Smith, M. (2023). *Coping with an Alzheimer's or dementia diagnosis - HelpGuide.org.* HelpGuide. https://www.helpguide.org/articles/alzheimers-dementia-aging/coping-with-an-alzheimers-or-dementia-diagnosis.htm

Robinson, L., Wayne, M., & Segal, J. (2018, November 2). *Alzheimer's and dementia care: Help for family caregivers.* HelpGuide. https://www.helpguide.org/articles/alzheimers-dementia-aging/tips-for-alzheimers-caregivers.htm

Rodriguez, D. (2021, May 11). *The importance of social interaction for those with Alzheimer's.* Tapestry Senior. https://www.tapestrysenior.com/2021/05/11/the-importance-of-social-interaction-for-those-with-alzheimers/

Rosenberger, P. (2017, September 13). *Rediscovering your identity as a caregiver.* The Caregiver Space. https://www.thecaregiverspace.org/rediscovering-your-identity-as-a-caregiver/

Sager, J. (2022, May 4). *100 caregiver affirmations to honor yourself and the amazing work you're doing.* Parade. https://parade.com/1373242/jessicasager/caregiver-affirmations/

Samuels, C. (2023, November 6). *Does insurance cover memory care? A detailed look at coverage and options.* A Place for Mom. https://www.aplaceformom.com/caregiver-resources/articles/does-insurance-cover-memory-care

Scallan, T. (2023, January 11). *How to remember our self-worth while caregiving.* Caregiving Experts. https://theultimatecaregivingexpert.com/how-to-remember-our-self-worth-while-caregiving/

Schempp, D. (2014, June 28). *When caregiving ends.* Family Caregiver Alliance. https://www.caregiver.org/resource/when-caregiving-ends/

Segal, J. (2018, December 27). *Hospice and palliative care - HelpGuide.org.* Https://HelpGuide. https://www.helpguide.org/articles/caregiving/hospice-and-palliative-care.htm

Serani, D. (2022, May 31). *Creating a caregiving self-care plan.* Psychology Today.

https://www.psychologytoday.com/us/blog/two-takes-depression/202205/
creating-caregiving-self-care-plan

Shapiro, S. (2011, May 24). *Rotating a schedule of care when looking after a loved-one.* Fifty plus Advocate. https://www.fiftyplusadvocate.com/2011/05/24/rotating-a-schedule-of-care-when-looking-after-a-loved-one/

Signs of dying in the elderly with dementia: End-stage. (n.d.). Cross Roads Hospice. https://www.crossroadshospice.com/hospice-resources/end-of-life-signs/dementia/

6 ways to handle family conflicts regarding a parent's care. (2022, August 3). Assisting Hands. https://assistinghands.com/50/how-to-address-family-disputes-about-parents-care/

6 ways to successfully communicate non-verbally with dementia residents. (2014, July 17). Linked Senior. https://www.linkedsenior.com/blog/2014/07/6-ways-to-successfully-communicate-non-verbally-with-dementia-residents/

Slatton, L. (2023, March 24). *Self care for the caregiver: 8 practical tips.* DailyCaring. https://dailycaring.com/self-care-for-the-caregiver-practical-tips/

Smebye, K. L., Kirkevold, M., & Engedal, K. (2012). How do persons with dementia participate in decision making related to health and daily care? A multi-case study. *BMC Health Services Research, 12*(1). https://doi.org/10.1186/1472-6963-12-241

Smith, M. (2019). *Caregiver stress and burnout.* Help Guide. https://www.helpguide.org/articles/stress/caregiver-stress-and-burnout.htm

Smith, M., Segal, J., & White, M. (2019, February 19). *Alzheimer's and dementia behavior management tips.* Help Guide. https://www.helpguide.org/articles/alzheimers-dementia-aging/alzheimers-behavior-management.htm

Soto-Rubio, A., Perez-Marin, M., Tomas Miguel, J., & Barreto Martin, P. (2018). Emotional distress of patients at end-of-life and their caregivers: Interrelation and predictors. *Frontiers in Psychology, 9.* https://doi.org/10.3389/fpsyg.2018.02199

Sreenivas, S. (2021, August 3). *What is grief counseling?* WebMD. https://www.webmd.com/balance/grief-counseling

Stokes, L. A., Combes, H., & Stokes, G. (2012). Understanding the dementia diagnosis: The impact on the caregiving experience. *Dementia, 13*(1), 59–78. https://doi.org/10.1177/1471301212447157

Stringfellow, A. (2019). *Activities for dementia patients: 50 tips and ideas to keep patients with dementia engaged.* Seniorlink. https://www.seniorlink.com/blog/activities-for-dementia-patients-50-tips-and-ideas-to-keep-patients-with-dementia-engaged

Swanson, D. (2019, February 21). *11 unique skills you need to become a caregiver.*

Caring Senior Service. https://www.caringseniorservice.com/blog/unique-skills-to-become-a-caregiver

Taking care of YOU: Self-care for family caregivers. (2023). Family Caregiver Alliance. https://www.caregiver.org/resource/taking-care-you-self-care-family-care givers/

Tay, C. (2022, May 4). *Building resilience in caregiving.* EHospice. https://ehospice.com/asia-pacific-posts/building-resilience-in-caregiving/

The benefits of self-forgiveness. (2019, August 2). Scope. https://scopeblog.stanford.edu/2019/08/02/the-benefits-of-self-forgiveness/

The important of routine and familiarity to persons with dementia. (2020, June 7). Alzheimer's Project. https://alzheimersproject.org/the-importance-of-routine-and-familiarity-to-persons-with-dementia/

The psychological and emotional impact of dementia. (2022, June 27). Alzheimer's Society. https://www.alzheimers.org.uk/get-support/help-dementia-care/understanding-supporting-person-dementia-psychological-emotional-impact

The three goodbyes. (2014, June 10). Fisher Center for Alzheimer's Research Foundation. https://www.alzinfo.org/pym/feature/the-three-goodbyes/

Top 10 caregiver tips for staying healthy and active. (2021a, October 25). American Heart Association. https://www.heart.org/en/health-topics/caregiver-support/top-10-caregiver-tips-for-staying-healthy-and-active

Top 16 caregiver apps for 2020. (2020, January 10). Where You Live Matters. https://www.whereyoulivematters.org/best-caregiver-apps/

Thurston, C. (2011, February 13). *Honoring the person within: Being there for a loved one with dementia.* Palliative & Supportive Care of Nantucket. https://www.pascon.org/resources-education/educational-articles/honoring-the-person-within-being-there-for-a-loved-one-with-dementia/

Understanding different types of dementia. (n.d.). National Institute on Aging. https://www.nia.nih.gov/health/alzheimers-and-dementia/understanding-different-types-dementia

Understanding how your relationship may change. (2022). Alzheimer Society of Canada. https://alzheimer.ca/en/help-support/i-have-friend-or-family-member-who-lives-dementia/understanding-how-your-relationship

Watson, S. (2022, January 11). *Caregiving help: Ask for what you need.* WebMD. https://www.webmd.com/alzheimers/alzheimers-caregiving-help

Wayne, M., Segal, J., & Robinson, L. (2019, June 11). *Late stage and end-of-life care.* Help Guide. https://www.helpguide.org/articles/end-of-life/late-stage-and-end-of-life-care.htm

Weber, T. (2016, March 9). *The mindset of a caregiver.* UK Human Resources. https://hr.uky.edu/thrive/03-09-2016/mindset-caregiver

Wei, M. (2018, October 17). *Self-care for the caregiver*. Harvard Health Blog. https://www.health.harvard.edu/blog/self-care-for-the-caregiver-2018101715003

Weigelt, M. (2022, March 18). *Dementia and living spaces- How to create a safe space*. Thrive USA Home Care. https://www.thriveusahomecare.com/dementia-and-living-spaces-how-to-create-a-safe-space/

What are palliative care and hospice care? (2021, May 14). National Institute on Aging. https://www.nia.nih.gov/health/hospice-and-palliative-care/what-are-pallia tive-care-and-hospice-care

What are the signs of end-stage dementia? (2023, October 18). Senior Services of America. https://seniorservicesofamerica.com/blog/what-are-the-signs-of-end-stage-dementia/

What types of insurance covers memory care costs? (2020, December 1). Copeland Oaks. https://www.copelandoaks.com/what-types-of-insurance-covers-memory-care-costs/

When people with dementia refuse help. (2009). Scie. https://www.scie.org.uk/demen tia/living-with-dementia/difficult-situations/refusing-help.asp

Why is routine important for dementia? (2020, July 27). Where You Live Matters. https://www.whereyoulivematters.org/importance-of-routines-for-dementia/

Wiederrich, D. (2023, October 6). *Factors to consider when evaluating Medigap coverage for dementia care*. Dementia Map. https://www.dementiamap.com/factors-to-consider-when-evaluating-medigap-coverage-for-dementia-care/

Woodruff, L. (2021, September 14). *Choosing the right long-term care facility*. AARP. https://www.aarp.org/caregiving/basics/info-2021/choosing-long-term-care-facility.html

Wright, K. (2021, December 7). *Forgiveness: A caregiver's hidden strength*. Seacare Homecare. https://www.seacarehomecare.com/resources/forgiveness-a-care givers-hidden-strength

Wynn, P. (2017, December). *How to reclaim life after years of caregiving*. Brain and Life. https://www.brainandlife.org/articles/reclaiming-life-after-years-of-care giving-is-a-gradual-up

Young, M. V. (2021, July 23). *Dementia and family dynamics*. Tender Rose. https://www.tenderrose.com/blog/all/dementia-family-dynamics

Your emotional reaction to the dementia diagnosis. (2021, September 7). Forward with Dementia. https://www.forwardwithdementia.org/en/article/2-1-your-emotional-reaction-to-the-dementia-diagnosis-being-told-someone-close-to-you-has-dementia-brings-up-strong-emotions/

Zagaria, M. A. (2013, May 21). *When communication becomes difficult: Is it dementia?* US Pharmacist. https://www.uspharmacist.com/article/when-communication-becomes-difficult-is-it-dementia

OpenAI. (2024). *ChatGPT* (4) [Large language model]. https://chat.openai.com